Hobart A. Burch, PhD

Basic Social Policy and Planning: Strategies and Practice Methods

Pre-publication
*REVIEWS,
COMMENTARIES,
EVALUATIONS . . .*

"At last! A social policy text that combines theory and practice knowledge with operational reality and wit to create the optimal learning tool. It is the current front-runner for initiating finishing undergraduate and beginning graduate students into the method and techniques of social policy processes.

Burch's career of social action, professional dedication, and intellectual contemplation has produced a publication that broadens the reader's interests while focusing learning on how to execute planning in the chaos, conflicts, and contradictions of current society. The foundations, approaches, and key elements are all there, with cogent examples. This is a truly useful book for social work education and related fields."

**Chauncey A. Alexander,
ACSW, LCSW, CAE**
*Professor/Instructor,
Department of Social Work,
California State University,
Long Beach, CA*

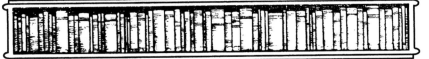

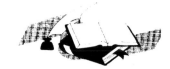

"**W**hat lifts this volume to a new level of interest and discourse on the subject of policy analysis and planning is the authoritative way in which the author illustrates and discusses the importance of making conscious use of the lively dialectical tension that is generated in the interaction of the five VIBES with the content of the six sequential planning steps.

Also new in this volume is a well-informed interdisciplinary perspective that includes economic theory, political science, social systems theory, history, and philosophy. The author's many years of experience within the federal government as well as in private and voluntary organizations yields a salty and exciting set of chapters in which a poignant relevance to the current policy dilemmas in the United States and Canada is immediately apparent to the reader."

Sheldon Rahn, DSW
*Founding Dean
and Emeritus Professor
of Social Policy and Social
Administration,
Wilfrid Laurier University,
Waterloo, Ontario*

"**D**rawing upon a wide range of academic disciplines and using stories, film, music, humor, and personal experience, Burch demystifies the planning process, making it both comprehensible and relevant to ordinary people as well as professional planners.

His treatment of values, interests, beliefs, ethics, and slants (VIBES) and their impact on planning decisions is especially well done and worthy of the attention of those endeavoring to teach policy analysis at any level. This book will be suitable for planning and policy courses across various disciplines."

Mari Ann Graham, MSW
*Assistant Professor,
School of Social Work,
University of St. Thomas,
St. Paul, MN*

"**B**asic Social Policy and Planning is a stimulating and thought-provoking treatment of an important subject. It is applicable to broad national issues and systematic social problems, as well as more limited agency and programmatic concerns. Burch examines and discusses the subject in depth in both philosophical and theoretical terms, but places greater emphasis on down-to-earth, concrete applications that are of practical value to practitioners.

The author distinguishes modern social planning with its value orientation from the purely mechanistic approaches of physical, engineering, and business planning from which it derives. Consequently, important elements of social planning are 'not easily defined or formulated.' Since decisions are often based on limited, inconclusive evidence, the author cautions the reader to be aware of the 'limitations of planning,' which could be a subtitle of this book.

Burch's work should appeal to a variety of audiences. Obviously, graduate students in social planning and policy development will find it most beneficial, as well as practitioners with program development and management responsibilities. Lastly, public officials should find the chapters on ethics and values informative."

Robert Langer, MS, ACSW
Planning and Development
Consultant, Philadelphia, PA

"**T**his is an especially useful basic text for planners, especially social welfare planners who are now drawn from many different disciplines. It offers a refreshingly different approach that simultaneously takes the mystery out of planning while also explaining the more complex tools of planning now used in public policy and political analyses, as well as in other fields such as business administration, engineering, architecture, and even in managing the personal affairs of daily life."

Robert Morris
Kirstein Professor Emeritus,
Brandeis University;
Cardinal Medeiros Lecturer,
University of Massachusetts,
Boston

More pre-publication
REVIEWS, COMMENTARIES, EVALUATIONS . . .

"**B**asic Social Policy and Planning is a book I should have read sixteen years ago when I first ran for public office. Planning is the missing link in 'crisis government' today. It is the process that can turn ideas into action, problems into solutions, and bring different agendas to consensus. The information in this book will help me become a more effective leader.

As Webster's dictionary has been a resource for effectively using the English language, this book will be a continual resource for setting policy. Section II, 'Different Approaches to Planning,' was of particular interest to me. One of the greatest challenges of public service is to be able to work on a daily basis with a wide variety of situations and personalities. Knowledge is power. The author has provided me with that knowledge."

(Hon.) Margaret B. Buhrmaster
Chairperson,
Schenectady County Legislature,
Schenectady, NY

The Haworth Press, Inc.

Basic Social Policy
and Planning
Strategies
and Practice Methods

HAWORTH Social Work Practice
Carlton E. Munson, DSW, Senior Editor

New, Recent, and Forthcoming Titles:

Basic Social Policy and Planning
Strategies and Practice Methods

Hobart A. Burch, PhD

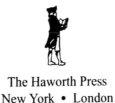

The Haworth Press
New York • London

The Haworth Press, Inc., 10 Alice Street, Binghamton, NY 13904-1580

Library of Congress Cataloging-in-Publication Data

Burch, Hobart A.
    Basic social policy and planning : strategies and practice methods / Hobart A. Burch.
       p.   cm.
    Includes bibliographical references and index.
    ISBN 0-7890-6026-4 (alk. paper)
    1. Social policy–Methodology. 2. Social planning–Methodology. I. Title.
HN28.B85 1996
361.6′1′01–dc20
                                                95-43400
                                                  CIP

To Jan Bast Burch, who has brought grace into my life and work, and who never stopped believing in this book. Although we are both congenital planners, our union was the most totally unplanned experience of our lives.

ABOUT THE AUTHOR

Hobart A. Burch, PhD, is Professor in the School of Social Work at the University of Nebraska where, as Director of the School of Social Work (1976-1981), he rebuilt the School's program and was successful in securing reaccreditation after reorganizing, increasing financial support, upgrading faculty standards, and revising curriculum. Prior to teaching, Dr. Burch held national leadership positions in the government, church, and charities sectors, including an appointment as Assistant to the U.S. Commissioner on Welfare. He is widely published in the areas of social welfare and social policy and is the author of *The Whys of Social Policy.*

CONTENTS

Foreword

The world today is characterized by societies and governments that confront a broad range of complex–and often interrelated–destructive social problems. Repeated frantic efforts to deal with this array of serious social problems have, at best, achieved only rare modest measures of improvement or success. These social problems, seemingly, yield neither to historic traditional approaches and interventions, nor to current ameliorative efforts in such pervasive problem areas as: inadequate public education systems; violent crime and delinquency phenomena; deteriorated marital and family stability; poor health services for very large populations at risk; alarming loss of respect for authority figures such as parents, teachers, policemen, or government officials and laws; and limited access to economic resources and economic opportunities for large critical populations.

The author, Dr. Hobart Burch, has conceptualized and elaborated a basic introduction to the nature of social policy analysis and planning development. He then presents a generic process of professional intervention and social work leadership that is required to achieve the planned improvement (i.e., the change goal) in the targeted chronic social problem's situation of concern. Such change efforts must have professional leaders who are endowed both with commitment to the goals of the change project, and with strong interpersonal skills essential to establishing and maintaining effective social relationships with many people who are located over a broad public and private spectrum of complexity.

This text is well conceptualized and interestingly developed, with the author drawing heavily upon a broad range of "classical literature" for many relevant quotations that admirably serve to trigger thought. Burch successfully weaves current practice experience illustrations into the text that are presented with critical insights and wry humor. This book serves very well as an introductory policy planning text in undergraduate programs and equally as a basic text in both graduate foundation sequences in social policy and in generic practice.

We are indebted to the author for providing a timely text that presents a comprehensive synthesis of theory and practice in basic policy analysis and strategic development processes and issues. He explores in depth the complex issues of *why?* and *what?* and *how?* related to attempts to deal constructively with serious social problems that characterize current society. This synthesis serves to guide and illuminate generic professional practice in the complex process aimed at effecting desirable social change and achieving improvement goals in a targeted social problem area of concern.

M. Mickey Lebowitz
Consultant, Professor Emeritus,
Fordham University Graduate
School of Social Service

ACKNOWLEDGMENTS

I wish to thank:

- Mickey Lebowitz, friend and mentor, without whose encouragement, counsel, and practical assistance this book would probably still be a draft in my computer.
- Jan Burch for editorial assistance at every stage. Her key function was to make sure it was interesting, readable, and clear.
- Bob Morris, from whom I learned policy and planning, for a critical review and assurance that it met his rigorous academic standards.
- Chauncey Alexander, for sharing the insights of a long career as a leader of his profession.
- My social policy and planning students over the years, for refining my perspectives in these related fields, and particularly my Spring 1995 social planning class, for serving as textbook guinea pigs and de facto reviewers of an earlier draft.
- University of Nebraska-Omaha, for a timely sabbatical.

I. FOUNDATIONS FOR ALL PLANNING

Planning *is*. You can't escape it. Life is a journey, a continuous series of trips from *here* (is) to *there* (will be). Whether as one individual, an organization, or a whole society, we exist within an array of currents and circumstances that are constantly moving and changing. If we want to have some control over this journey, we must decide where we want to end up (goals) and how to go there–or at least part way (course of action).

The alternative is a *vagabond model* ("a wandering from place to place without settled habitation"). Drift with the current, taking your chances on where it may lead you. Plankton does this (and often ends up in the belly of a goal-directed whale). This is a perfectly legitimate philosophy, existentialism. However, most of us, most of the time, prefer to have something to say about it.

Chapter 1 offers an overview of the immensely diverse area of "planning," a basic generic model, and, in fairness, the rationales for not planning.

There is no single consensus model of *the* proper way to plan. In real life, each plan is unique, tailored to the particular situation, with a blend of approaches and techniques. How do you talk about it if it is never quite the same twice? Some classical music etudes offer a half-dozen variations on a theme. The basic model used here is the unadorned "theme." The remainder of the book is variations on it.

No one operates in a vacuum. All planning is guided, consciously or unwittingly, explicitly or implicitly, openly or covertly by a set of VIBES: where you and "they" are coming from, both literally and figuratively: Values, Interests, Beliefs, Ethics, and Slant.

Chapter 2 addresses value choices, interests, beliefs about what the world is really like, and other slants. Chapter 3 picks up on ethical considerations, particular in relation to distributional justice,

1

whether the end justifies the means, and ways to decide a mixed bag of good and bad in gray-area ethics.

Chapters 4 and 5 demonstrate how different beliefs and ways of thinking affect one's view of reality, which in turn dramatically limits and colors the planning decisions. Chapter 4 contrasts the planning implications of one's worldview and systems model. A Newtonian physics view of the world as a predictable mechanism carries very different planning implications from a social systems theory modeled on a living organism. The same is true for our view of what people and society are really like (*Weltanschauung*). Our approach will be affected by whether we see the setting as a predatory jungle, a benign fellowship, or a corporate body that transcends individual interests.

Chapter 5 explores how the way we think affects what we look for, how we look for it, what we actually see, how we process it, and the conclusions we draw. Our intake approaches include the scientific method, the clinical method, heuristic trial and error, and experiential intuition-insight. Bounded (narrowly confined) and non-bounded (open-ended) rationality each have their proper place. A broad dilemma for any planning is how to reduce impossibly complex situations to manageable proportion without losing important data and insight–and how we draw conclusions from what we see.

Chapter 1

Introduction:
What is Planning?

*My interest is in the future
because I am going to spend the rest of my life there.*

–C. F. Kettering

*There is nothing permanent except change.
You can't step in the same river twice.*

–Heraclitus

TO PLAN

I finished high school early and went away to college, leaving my hometown and all my school friends. When I came back for Christmas, everything seemed the same, except that I was no longer part of it. I felt nostalgia for the solid, stable, comfortable world I had left.

> I know a tear would glisten
> If once more I could listen
> To that gang that sang "Heart of My Heart."

–*B. Ryan, 1926*

Ten years later all but one of the old gang has dispersed to seek their fortunes in California, Kansas, New Jersey, and other exotic places. The typewriter factory closed, and laid-off workers moved away. A high-tech business moved in, bringing new folks with different life styles. Had I stayed put I would be in a different place anyway.

Life is a continuous journey from here (is) to there (will be), in a river where currents and circumstances are constantly moving and changing. Since all of our "heres" are moving too, we cannot avoid going to some "there." Your only choice is whether you "go with the flow" wherever the drift takes you or, by planning, take a hand in it.

What Is Planning?

My dictionary* says planning is "any method of thinking out actions or purposes beforehand." It is deciding where you want to go (your "there") and how to get there from here.

Koontz and O'Donnell (1972, p. 113) offer a more elaborate definition:

> Planning is deciding in advance what to do, how to do it, when to do it, and who is to do it. Planning bridges the gap from where we are to where we want to go. It makes it possible for things to occur which would not otherwise happen. Although the exact future can seldom be predicted and factors beyond control may interfere with the best-laid plans, without planning events are left to chance. Planning . . . is the conscious determination of a course of action, the basing of decisions on purpose, facts, and considered estimates.

Planning is *future oriented*. It is something you want to get to. It assumes that the future is sufficiently predictable to act.

It is *proactive*, taking initiative to change things, either to solve a problem or exploit an opportunity.

Planning itself is a dynamic, fluid *process not a product*. It

---

*Unless otherwise noted, definitions that are given throughout this book are from the following standard dictionaries:
The American College Dictionary. (NY: Random House, 1970).
Webster's New 20th Century Dictionary of the English Language, 2nd Edition. (NY: World Publishing Co., 1971).

usually produces draft road maps or blueprints along the way. As the planning process continues, these draft "plans" are updated, revised, and reprinted as needed. "Planners tend to forget too often that the map is not the terrain" (Hudson 1979, pp. 392-93).

Planning uses conscious, organized, *rational analysis* to size up the situation, choose goals and objectives, and select doable means. However, while the *process* is analytical, the *information* it uses includes direct experience, intuition, insight, and common sense along with systematic scientific data.

It is closely related to three other "P's":

- A *policy* is "any governing principle, plan, or course of action." Policy planning is development of an overall framework for specific plans. This incorporates such areas as beliefs and values, mission, long term goals, boundaries, and rules. It is sometimes called strategic planning.
- A *program* is "an outline of work to be done; a pre-arranged plan of procedure." Program planning is development of medium-to short-range objectives and the means to carry them out. This is sometimes called tactical planning. (In administration, it can also mean an ongoing mechanism to carry out a set of activities within the policy framework.)
- A *project* is "a unique piece of work having a finite life and producing an identifiable product or achieving a specific aim on time and within specified resource limits" (Canada, 1982, p. 82). Project planning is the nitty-gritty of achieving a concrete objective.

Where Is Planning?

Planning is applicable to all areas of life, large and small, long term or short, societal or individual. For instance, my own planning efforts have variously included:

- A Department of Labor youth work training program.
- Grocery shopping for the coming week.
- Attaining gender equality for clergy in a mainline denomination.
- Building a cottage on Cape Cod.

- A large corporation's program for philanthropy and community support.
- Assuring adequate personal retirement income.
- A mandatory national program-accounting standard for social agencies.
- A trip from Omaha to the Florida Keys.
- Rebuilding a graduate professional school to regain its accreditation.
- Helping a graduate student design her own tailored Plan of Study.
- Writing this book.

WHO PLANS

Many fields and professions claim planning as their own. They are all correct, for planning belongs to each and is the special province of no single one.

Official Planning Fields

An early entrant into "modern" planning was public physical planning, perhaps dating from Britain's "city beautiful" planning of model garden suburbs in 1893. By the 1920s, "master planning" had taken root in Chicago. The parent disciplines were architecture and engineering. Today this is called "urban and regional" planning in the United States and "location" planning in Britain. Over time, it has expanded its boundaries from housing to include transportation and the entire physical infra (underlying) structure of an area, the natural environment, and social impacts of physical planning.

Meanwhile, on a parallel track, business, especially large industry, embarked on an engineering-based "scientific management" road in the early twentieth century. This eventually evolved into a cost benefit production planning model. In 1961, it was brought by a business executive, Robert McNamara, to the Department of Defense as "PPBS" (Program Planning and Budgeting System) and quickly spread across the spectrum of domestic programs as well.

Although much of it was officially rescinded by a later administration, cost benefit analysis has continued to expand in traditional physical, business, human services, and military planning.

A third parallel planning track involved collaborative planning among human services. It began in 1869 with the first Charity Organization Society in London and progressed to Community Chests and Councils of Social Agencies. Its best known practitioners today are United Ways and Jewish Federations. The primary discipline is a branch of social work, called variously "social administration," "community organization," and "macro practice," which has been taught at the graduate degree level since 1901. It has emphasized informed collaborative decision making and coordination more than the paternalistic expertise approach preferred by the technical planning disciplines.

Influenced by the popular growth of sociology and psychology, the collaborative planning approach emerged in business in the 1920s as part of a human relations school of administration, which focused on employee motivation. It is sometimes called industrial psychology. These have blended into a number of participatory business planning models. A recent popular one has been Total Quality Management (TQM), a grandchild of W. Edwards Deming, who mobilized the United States industrial war in World War II. When his methods were rebuffed by postwar American business, he took them to Japan, as a consultant in rebuilding their economy, from which they were exported to the United States a generation later.

Meanwhile, public human services emerged piecemeal in the early 1900s in Britain and the 1930s in the United States. After World War II, Britain and most other industrial nations embarked on comprehensive social infrastructure planning, called the Welfare State, to complement the physical infrastructure already subject to comprehensive public planning. (The United States rejected this in favor of an approach popularly known as "disjointed incrementalism.")

Macro (economy-wide) economic planning languished in capitalist countries because of antiplanning free market ideology, which remains strong on rhetoric if not in practice today. The severe economic crises of the 1920s and 1930s opened the door to broad planned interventions, derived from theories of John Maynard Keynes, using broad fiscal and monetary mechanisms.

Targeted economic development planning emerged from other crises. In Russia, the Revolution led to economic Five Year Plans, which achieved some limited successes despite crude technical and administrative limitations. It was more effective in rebuilding economies crippled by World War II. Ironically, although the United States was an initiating partner in this through the MacArthur occupation of Japan and the Marshall Plan in Europe, targeted economic development never quite caught on at home.

Last but far from least, the military have developed what may be the most sophisticated comprehensive rational planning system of all, using game theory and simulation as well as administrative planning methods developed in business.

While many of these sophisticated models are products of the computer age, planning is not new to the military field. At Thermopylae in 480 B.C., 300 Spartans, through the wise tactical planning of General Leonidas, blocked a Persian army reported to be 2.6 million, while, as reported by Herodotus in 450 B.C., loser Xerxes ignored his uncle's counsel, "Take my advice and do not run any such terrible risk when there is no necessity to do so. . . . Nothing is more valuable to a man than to lay his plans carefully and well" (Herodotus, *The Histories*, ea. 446 B.C.).

Planning Professionals

In addition to academic programs which call themselves "planning," planners seem to emerge regularly from many related fields and disciplines, including:

- Architecture
- Business Administration
- Economics
- Education
- Engineering
- Military Science
- Political Science and Policy Analysis
- Public Administration

- Social change programs, such as the Industrial Areas Foundation
- Social Work
- Sociology

Personal Life

Perhaps the number one planning area is "none of the above," not the big leagues but the sandlots of ordinary life.

We all need basic planning skills because we are planning constantly in large and small ways in our daily lives. There are broad- and long-range plans, such as building a career, providing for our children's future, preparing for retirement. There are middle-sized plans, such as planning one's college program, developing a research project, winning the league championship, or regaining proper fitness. There are baby bear projects, the foot soldiers of our lives, such as a triptik itinerary, a term paper, or setting the week's menu.

A BASIC PLANNING MODEL

There is no single consensus model of the proper way to plan. In real life, each plan is unique, tailored to the particular situation, with a blend of approaches and techniques. How do you talk about it if it is never quite the same twice? As a point of reference for later discussions on the ingredients and variations of planning, below is a generic rational planning model which I have given the acronym, BASIC: *Broad Analysis, Strategy, and Incremental Choices*. Our "solution" is a basic, generic model. Some classical music etudes offer a half-dozen variations on a theme. This model is the unadorned "theme." The remainder of the book is variations on it.

The model is *eclectic*, drawing upon diverse approaches and techniques:

> You take a leg from some old table;
> You take an arm from some old chair;
> You take a neck from some old bottle,

And from a horse you take some hair.
Then you put them all together
With a piece of string and glue,
And I'll get more [planning] from that [gosh darn] dummy
Than I ever got from you! (Old college song)

Said Cervantes, "The proof of the pudding is in the eating." The validity of a planning model is not in its logical beauty or symmetry. It is a tool, no more, no less; a means not an end in itself. Its merit is the extent to which it accomplishes its sole reason for being: to figure out where to go and then to get there.

Although the BASIC model, summarized here and elaborated in Chapters 9 through 11, can be followed with good effect, one size does not fit all. Adapt it to your style and the particular planning task. Use your own terminology. Elaborate further for complex planning, condense for simpler tasks. Keep what is helpful. Skip what is not. Revise what is adaptable. Substitute or add whatever fits better.

RECURRING DIALECTIC THEMES

Dialectic examines a situation from two different points of view. An early model is the Socratic and Platonic give-and-take dialogue. Another is the traditional Talmudic "on the one hand . . . on the other hand" approach to interpreting Jewish Law.

The modern version, developed in the early 1800s by Georg Wilhelm Friedrich Hegel, has three steps:

1. *Thesis* (Greek for "position") is the starting point, "a proposition to be maintained or defended in argument."
2. *Antithesis* is "an opposing or contrasting position." Hegel says that every thesis contains the seeds of its anti-thesis.
3. *Synthesis* is "the putting of two or more things together so as to form a whole."

In planning, there are inherent dialectical tensions that recur at nearly every stage.

One is between *normative and empirical*. A norm is "a standard." Normative refers to establishing such norms and applying them to choices about what is desirable or not. Its sources are many. Obviously, one is the *a priori values and beliefs* of the planner, both conscious and unwitting. Another is what is *mandated* by forces beyond the planner's control, such as legal authority, power elites, plan sponsors, vested interests, culture, the state of the economy, or weather. A third source is participative, based on *preferences* of those to be affected. While it receives much lip service, a good hard normative look is often neglected in practice.

Empirical refers to observed "facts" about the situation and inferences based on them. These facts relate to conditions, what caused them, and what realistically can or cannot be done. A synthesis of normative and empirical helps the planner to select the best combination of desirability and effectiveness.

Another dialectic is between *yin and yang*. The latter represents a no-nonsense focus on concrete action, conflict, control. By itself it may be a ship without a navigator.

The yin perspective is more intuitive and experiential. It offers broader and deeper perspectives. It absorbs and accommodates to intangible qualitative, aesthetic, emotional, and spiritual elements. By itself it may be a guru in an ivory tower. A synthesis can be a well-built ship *with* a navigator. In a balanced plan, there is a clear sense of mission and direction carried out through a practical, well-organized course of action.

A *third dialectic* is between the established plan and feedbacks which diverge from what was projected. The synthesis is periodic adaptive revisions of the plan.

SIX STAGES OF PLANNING

The BASIC model is a framework which organizes a complex and confusing subject area. It has six functionally sequential levels, from the most general to the most concrete:

1. *Global vision* perspective
2. *Strategic* planning
3. *Tactical* planning
4. *Operational* design

5. *Implementation* activity
6. *Evaluation* review

Global Vision Perspective

First, determine your area of interest: what, where, who, and why? Goals and targets will be within this boundary. Whatever is outside is dealt with to the extent that it affects, or is affected by, the plan.

In relation to this area, explore your own values, interests, beliefs, ethics, and slants, as well as those of others who will affect, or be affected by, the plan. Many of them are a priori (before the fact), coloring perceptions of reality, truth, good and bad. They *always* operate, whether we know it or not. Anyone who claims to be "value-neutral" or "interest-free" is either lying or unaware.

Within this context, develop a broad perspective on:

1. What *is:* the *existing situation.*
2. What *should be:* the *desirable situation,* your ultimate, ideal destination. Why? (Compromises come later on.)

Strategic Planning

Having identified the existing situation, what is desirable, and criteria for setting priorities, the next step is to explore the discrepancy between "is" and "should be." The purpose of this stage is to select goals that will contribute toward filling this *gap.* This involves:

- What: *needs assessment.* What are the unmet needs and/or the unachieved opportunities?
- Why: *diagnosis* of the gap. What are its causes in past or present policies, actions, defaults, barriers?
- Where: *key results areas* (KRA) where significant contributions can be made toward filling or crossing the gap.
- Whither ("to what place"): *long-range goals* for each KRA, from which are developed *middle-range goals* for this specific planning project.

Tactical Planning

Within the plan's goal, choose the first leg on the trip, a specific time-limited objective along with the means by which to do it. Steiner (1979, p. 22) calls this "tactical planning . . . courses of action used to implement strategic plans."

Operational Design

Next lay out, step-by-step, who does what, when, with what resources. Key steps along the way, called *milestones*, are designated to mark progress within the design. This is variously called programming, project management, or operational planning. It may use such techniques as critical path networking, Gantt charts, and flow charts. Included in the activities are sequencing of tasks, assuring resources, and scheduling.

Implementation Activity

At this point we may be crossing the gray area between planning and administration. It doesn't really matter what you call it. By any name it is actually doing it. In a large plan, delegation of tasks and responsibilities are finalized, along with standards for evaluation and lines of accountability and supervision. In a micro plan, all that may be needed is for you to carry it out personally.

In all plans, an appropriate system to *monitor* progress and performance is set up, usually built around the milestones. It is also desirable to have some system of monitoring external assumptions (about factors you don't control) to get early warning of possible later problems. Minor preventive or corrective adjustments are made to adapt to unexpected circumstances. A feedback channel is set up to enable "higher" levels to respond to major problems that cannot be resolved at the "line" level.

Evaluation Review

Both for your own satisfaction and to make your boss or constituency happy, you want to know how well you succeeded and whether it was worth the cost. A socially responsible planner includes significant side effects. If possible, design the evaluation also to address cause and effect hypotheses, comparing the relative effectiveness of different approaches.

Another key benefit of evaluation is *feedback* for future thinking and planning. If it is built into the monitoring system described above, it may improve midstream revisions in the current plan as well.

LIMITATIONS OF THE MODEL

Like all models, BASIC is simplified. The actual process is more variable. In a complex plan, levels three and four might be broken down into any number of increasingly specific sublevels.

At the opposite extreme, in a very simple plan, a concrete objective may be also be its strategic goal.

These stages can be portrayed as a conventional top-down model, or perhaps laid on its side to show logical left-to-right progression from "first cause" to "final action."

Of course, that is not how our minds really work in practice. An accurate model would show a plethora of arrows running up, down, and sideways all over the place as our minds jump around. Or perhaps it would resemble the board game, "Snakes and Ladders." You follow a path that winds back and forth up the hill. If you land on a space with a ladder, you climb it as a shortcut to the next level. If you land on a snake, you slide down its back to an earlier level. However, it is immensely helpful to hark back regularly to the logical structure to renew our perspective and be sure we haven't overlooked something important in our wanderings.

GENERAL OBSERVATIONS ON THE MODEL

There is a hierarchy of interlocking ends and means within the overall planning framework. Each level's ends are subdivided into several subends at the next level, from the most global "desirable situation" down to a specific task. Looking "upward," each lower-level end is a means toward achieving the next higher level's end. For instance, completing library research is a task-end . . . which is a means toward the subobjective end of completing a term paper . . . which is a means toward the objective of credit for the course . . . which is a means toward the middle-range goal of earning a degree . . . which is a means toward a long-range professional career goal. Steiner (1979, p. 22) observes:

> Planning decisions range along a spectrum from strategies at one end to tactics at the other. . . . At the extremes there are clear distinctions between the two, but when they move closer to one another they become indistinguishable. Also, it should be noted that what may be a tactic to a chief executive officer may be a strategy to a subordinate.

Time dimensions vary with the level. While there are no hard and fast rules, conventional times tend to fall within the following ranges:

- Global vision of the desirable situation: unlimited.
- Strategic long-term mission goal: ten to thirty years.
- Strategic middle range plan goal: three to five years.
- Specific objective-means tactical plan: one year or less.
- Operational design, each task: hours, days, or weeks.

The process is semirepetitive. One way or another, whether quick and dirty, comprehensive, or somewhere in between, each level repeats the process of identifying alternatives, evaluating them, and selecting the most suitable one(s). However, the basis for rating varies with the level. At the higher levels where direction and perspective are needed, there is more weight given to normative, intangible, and holistic aspects. As we approach the concrete action stage, these choices have already been made, and the focus shifts increasingly to concrete practical feasibility elements.

Planning skills vary with the levels too. Intuitive insight and broad vision are assets at the broad levels, whereas technical skills and specialized expertise become more important at the lower levels. In large plans, it is not uncommon to have different folk working at the different levels, tied together by formal lines of delegation and (hopefully) informal relationships of sharing and trust. In a small project one person must be a general practitioner.

Partial Planning

While a plan is not complete without all six levels, there are many models and approaches that involve only partial planning. This is quite appropriate in many circumstances, provided someone else has already done the higher-prior stages one way or another or, in the opposite direction, someone will pick up the later stages where you left off.

In its original incarnation, strategic planning was a partial model developed in the corporate business field, which already had technically competent but disjointed tactical planning. It was a corrective that *added* an integrative broad perspective at the top management level. (In later versions, the definition of "strategic planning" was broadened to include all BASIC levels.)

At the other end of the line, Project Management is partial planning at the operational design and implementation levels. It is called upon only after the strategic and tactical plans have been decided.

FAILING TO PLAN

Would you like to swing on a star
And be better off than you are . . .
Or would you rather be a pig? . . .
If you don't care a feather or a fig,
You may grow up to be a pig.

–Johnny Burke, 1944
"Swinging on a Star"

There are lots of ways not to do rational planning. According to the song, you can be a pig or a mule or a fish instead—at a price. One way is to be *passive*. Accept the status quo. Go with the flow. "If it ain't broke, don't fix it." This probably means settling for less than what it could be and deferring to somebody else's preferences. It is often associated with feelings of depression, alienation, and/or powerlessness.

The other extreme is to be impulsive. Some impulsive actions work out very well. (They have certainly spiced up my marriage.) More often, when we fail to think things through, we do a vast project in a half-vast way: inefficient, unreliable, and error prone.

We can avoid the effort of planning by being *obsessive*, dealing with each item large or small as it comes up without priority or anticipation. This ain't all bad! In a national church office, after returning from an especially long and exhausting field trip, I sometimes allowed two days for obsessiveness. The first day back, after putting out any urgent fires, I was available to all staff on any matter on a first come, first served basis. The second day, I stayed home and went through my in-box stack doggedly from top to bottom, measuring progress by the inch. On the third day I rose again, re-energized for creative planning and leadership.

In a popular cartoon, two nebbishes slumped inertly in their chairs, feet outstretched on the coffee table, are saying "One of these days we've just got to get organized." Without the organizing benefit of planning, we often fritter away time, energy, money, potential. Our decisions are disjointed. We consider the next action only after the previous action is completed. Bob Harlan, former executive of the National YMCA, once observed to me in conversation, "Anyone can manage by objective. It takes a genius to manage by crisis!"

NONPLANNING PHILOSOPHIES

Responsible people may conscientiously oppose planning. You don't have to buy their whole argument to benefit from wisdom and insights which may enrich your life through "selective nonplanning."

Existentialism

Existentialism is "a philosophy of nihilism and pessimism which holds that each man exists as an individual in a purposeless universe." A classic Peggy Lee song expressed it:

Is that all there is?
If that's all there is, my friend, then let's keep dancing;

Let's break out the booze and have a ball,
If that's all-l-l there is.

–J. Lieber and M. Stoller, 1966
"Is That All There Is?"

Existentialism dismisses natural law and any systems theory. The here-and-now is all there is. There is no consistency on which to predict the future, a precondition for planning. Even if there were, you can't plan without a goal. With no purpose and no destination, there can be no goals. All we can do is cope.

A less gloomy version of existentialism is the Ecclesiastes proverb, "A man has no better thing under the sun than to eat, to drink, and to be merry."

Determinism

All things are determined by fate–or by predestination–or by Allah's will–or by the inexorable dialectic of history. "While determinists differ about the nature of the determining causes," explains Kohl (1992, p. 60), "no matter what the cause, a view is deterministic if it denies the possibility that the world could be other than it is." Obviously, planning is useless.

After the disillusionments of the Depression and the War, the optimistic religious humanism of the Social Gospel was succeeded by a "neo-orthodox" return to a pessimistic view of inadequacy and dependency upon the grace of God to achieve anything at all. My seminary classmates "revised" a social gospel hymn (W. P. Merrill, 1911) to fit the new "spin." The old version:

Rise up oh men of God;
His kingdom tarries long.
Bring in the day of brotherhood,
And end the night of wrong.

Our determinist version:

Sit down oh men of God;
His kingdom *He* will bring,

But what or where or when or how:
You cannot do a thing!

Natural Law – Western Style

François Quesnay, an eighteenth-century physician and physiologist, observed that a natural balancing of forces within the body did a better job of maintaining health and restoring equilibrium without the interventions of physicians, who subverted the natural functions with their bleedings, potions, and leeches. Calling himself a Physiocrat, he inferred his physiological premises to society at large. One might describe this outlook as saying the economy will remain healthier if you let it take its natural course rather than meddle. He coined the phrase, "*laissez faire*," which means "leave it alone to do its own thing."

A few years later, this became a cornerstone of Adam Smith's market economics. The natural law of supply and demand naturally maintains a cyclical equilibrium in which movement away from a balance between demand and supply automatically triggers millions of independent counteractions which restore equilibrium, analogous to the body triggering insulin to lower high blood sugar and giving runners "second wind" by releasing reserves to restore a depleted blood sugar level. It opposes any kind of central planning or control which interferes with this natural function. By definition, the free market has no predetermined future goals. Results are known only ex post facto (after the fact).

Charles Darwin observed that evolution occurred through survival of the best-adapted to whatever environment they were in. Herbert Spencer projected this into Social Darwinism, which concluded that no "artificial" (planned) intervention in society should interfere with God's natural law: "The unfit must be eliminated as nature intended, for the principle of natural selection must not be violated by the artificial preservation of those least able to take care of themselves" (Trattner, 1989, p. 83).

Joan Robinson (1960, p. 2) is skeptical about these neat and orderly laws of nature:

> The course which is best for each individual to pursue his own interests is rarely the same as the course best calculated to

promote interests of society as a whole, and if its economic system appears somewhat fantastic or even insane—as when foodstuffs are destroyed while men go hungry—we must remember that it is not surprising that the interaction of free individual decisions should lead so often to irrational, clumsy, and bewildering results.

Natural Law – Eastern Style

Tao is "the way." In Taoism, nature is a continuous dynamic interplay between forces, as opposed to the structural, mechanistic systems of classical Western science. However, we can find some Western parallels. An early one is the philosophy of Heraclitus (ca. 500 B.C.), who may have been influenced by Eastern thought. "All is flux, nothing is stationary." It has reentered Western worldviews by way of the theory of relativity and quantum physics.

In the world of Tao, movement is cyclical, going out from and returning to balance through a blending of counterforces. Returning is the motion of Tao. Going far means returning. To understand this circular world concept, imagine going in a straight line north from the equator. Eventually (after reaching the North Pole) you will find yourself going back toward the equator.

In Taoism, the polar forces are *yin* and *yang*. Yang is proactive; yin is receptive and contemplative. Yang exerts overt power; yin is yielding. *King* is the symbol of yang; yin's is *Sage*. A Western parallel may be the motto engraved over the entrance to my junior high school:

> Knowledge is proud that he has learn'd so much.
> Wisdom is humble that he knows no more.

> *—Cowper, 1785*

A blended harmony of yin and yang is desired. Taoism stresses the yin side. It is better to have too little than too much, to leave things undone than to overdo them. "The sage avoids excess, extravagance and indulgence (Lao Tzu, *Tao Te Ching*)." Intuitive intelligence transcends rational analysis. Action follows the natural order when it is a spontaneous response to that insight.

Taoism includes a concept of "nonaction" called *wu-wei*, which is refraining from activity contrary to nature, a principle we have already encountered in the origins of *laissez faire* and Social Darwinism. "Nonaction does not mean doing nothing and keeping silent. Let everything be allowed to do what it naturally does, so that its nature will be satisfied" (Chuang Tzu, quoted in Needham, 1956).

Romanticism

Romanticism emphasizes feelings, imagination, inspiration, and natural spontaneity, transcending the tunnel vision of materialistic technical and economic analysis.

> The world is too much with us; late and soon,
> Getting and spending, we lay waste our powers;
> Little we see in Nature that is ours;
> We have given our hearts away, a sordid boon . . .
> For this, for everything, we are out of tune;
> It moves us not.

> *—Wordsworth, 1806*

If the poets' lines touch us, there must be a place in our lives to "wander lonely as a cloud" or, with Tennyson, to contemplate a "flower in a crannied wall." Let's start now! Take a deep breath, let it out slowly, and savor this obvious nonplanning situation:

> Cruising down the river on a Sunday afternoon,
> The sun above, the one you love, waiting for the moon . . .
> The birds above all sing of love, a gentle sweet refrain;
> The winds around all make a sound like softly falling rain.

> *—Emily Beadell, 1945*
> "Cruising Down the River"

Planning Creeps in Anyway

Our song above continues:

> Just two of us together, we'll **PLAN** our honeymoon,
> Cruising down the river on a Sunday afternoon.

Oops! We said the P word! Can't we get away from it anywhere? Maybe Taoism is right: going out is coming back. Planning in its place enables nonplanning romanticism in its place. Most honeymoons are not idyllic. Perhaps you should plan what, where, and how to assure that yours will be more so. As I gaze out across the ocean from my seaside vacation home, the view is romantic, especially at sunset. However, this did not happen by chance on a teacher's salary. As the old bank ads said, "Wishing won't do it, saving will"–plus a lot of planning over a period of many years.

Perhaps people have a natural instinct to be proactive. Free market economics deters only some kinds of planning. Within it, entrepreneurs plan like crazy to beat the system and their competition. When they face recessions, they are not content to let natural law take its slow course. They clamor for government-planned countercyclical strategies. If they get strong enough, they aspire to centralized planning and control of their market.

Predestinarian Calvinists believed in absolute determinism, yet do you know any group that was more prudently plan-driven and controlling than the Puritans? They did their damnedest (literally) to help God along.

So did my "sit down, oh men of God" seminary classmates. They did not withdraw to monasteries and "let God do it." They shared a deep nonrational commitment to making this a better world. Instead of deterring them, low expectations gave their activism high frustration tolerance and staying power by immunization against disappointment. When you expect little, you are "surprised by joy" and sustained by even small or temporary successes. And then, like the Puritans, they believed we must prevail eventually because we are instruments of God's will. The same pattern may be seen in supposedly fatalistic Muslims, and in Marxists who profess a doctrine of historical determinism.

Why did Taoists stress the wu-wei yin? Was it in fact a matter of restoring the balance in a world dominated by yang? "What the world needs *now* is love, sweet love. That's the only thing there's just too little of."

These nonplanning worldviews have an important contribution to make to rational planning, which we will discuss in later chapters. They can provide major qualitative, intangible, insightful, and perhaps inspirational "data" inputs to complement (not replace) the quantified "facts" to which much of planning restricts itself. This is particularly important at the global and strategic levels of setting planning direction.

On the other hand, if that's all there is, then let's keep dancing.

REFERENCES

Canada Government: Regional and Economic Expansion (1982). *Project management handbook*. Ottawa.

Cowper, W. (1785), "The task." In Bartlett, J., *Familiar quotations,* 13 ed. (1955), p. 364. Boston: Little Brown & Co.

Herodotus (450 BC), *The Histories*, Book VII, 1972 edition. London: Penguin Books, p. 447.

Hudson, B. (1979). "Comparisons of current planning theories." *Journal of the American Institute of Planners*, 45, pp. 387-398.

Kohl, H.(1992). *From archetype to zeitgeist*. Boston: Little Brown.

Koontz, H. and O'Donnell, C. (1972). *Principles of management: An analysis of managerial functions*. 5th ed. New York: McGraw Hill.

Lao Tzu. (1973). *Tao Te Ching* (Ch. 26). Translated by Ch'u Ta Kao. New York: Samuel Weisner.

Needham, J. (1956). *Science and civilization in China, Vol. II*. Cambridge, England: Cambridge University Press, pp. 68-69.

Robinson, J. (1960). *Introduction to the theory of employment*. New York: St. Martin's.

Steiner, G. (1979). *Strategic planning*. New York: Free Press.

Trattner, W. (1989). *From poor law to welfare state*. 4th ed. New York: Free Press.

Chapter 2

Getting in Touch with Our VIBES

We find reasons for what we want to do.
Men desire first, then they reason.

–Walter Lippmann
A Preface to Politics, 1913

VIBES

All planning choices reflect where the actors are coming from, both literally and figuratively. Good planning is aware of, and makes thoughtful choices about, its **VIBES**:

- *Values:* "a criterion for deciding desirability."
- *Interests:* "in respect to advantage or detriment."
- *Beliefs:* "acceptance of something as true."
- *Ethics*: "standards of conduct and moral judgment."
- *Slants*: "a particular tendency or inclination, especially one which prevents unprejudiced consideration of a question."

There are pitfalls in uncritical acceptance of VIBES as "given." Unwitting planners may assume that their VIBES are universal or at least a consensus of those who will affect or be affected by the plan. In small projects this may be true. However, in any broad social, economic, military, physical, or corporate planning, it is a bit naive to think so.

It is normal for subordinates to accept VIBES dictated by authority in such forms as legislation, canon law, an agency mission statement, or delegation from a superior. This is okay, as long as they understand that their "signing on" makes them coaccountable for the consequences. Few of us accept Eichmann's rationale that he was guiltless when he slaughtered a million Jews and Slavs because he was merely following Hitler's orders.

VALUES AND INTERESTS

Values

A *value* is an *a priori* belief about what is good, right, or desirable. Values are often rooted in beliefs about religion, natural law, and human rights: "We hold these truths to be self-evident . . . ." They are installed in our mental "program" by our culture of origin, just as we install default programs in our computers. Like the computer program, we customize our values in response to life experience and particular circumstances.

As the ultimate criteria for defining well-being and harm, gains and losses, benefits and costs, values have an overwhelming impact on planning.

Test this out yourself. Consider two values, both widely professed in our society: (1) the guiding value in most social planning is economic: "the almighty dollar, that great object of universal devotion throughout our land" (Irving, 1856), and (2) a majority of Americans also profess a religion whose founder explicitly rejects this in favor of a spiritual value: "You cannot serve God and mammon" (Matthew 6:24). Sit for a moment and let your imagination lay out a life career plan based on value #1. Now, redraw the career plan using value #2. A tad different?

You can analyze values rationally to be clear what they are. You can know where they came from by tracing them back step by step to a first premise. You can evaluate the consistency of an applied value with its professed premise. You can freely criticize other people's values against the standard of your own a priori beliefs. You can debate the merits of conflicting values. You can change them.

What you *can't* do is prove or disprove them empirically, for science can measure only that which is material.

There may be an Absolute Truth. Some claim to possess it. They don't. Others say there is no such thing in the first place.

Paul offers a middle ground between absolutism and relativism with his limited claim to "the light of revelation . . . *but we have this treasure in earthenware pots*" (II Corinthians 4:7). We can get a pretty good working model of Truth and Good for our plan by examining values with *bold humility*. The boldness is to go with the best you can come up with. Whatever its deficiencies, it should be better than blind groping, drawing straws, or cynical self-serving. The humility is remembering that it is carried in a clay pot, and remaining open to better pots if they emerge along the way.

Interests

In finance, interest is the money gained from lending it. More broadly, an *interest* is any gain or other advantage for a particular individual, organization, or collective group, All plans promote somebody's interest. Otherwise, why do it? Many plans may also subvert someone else's interest through harmful side effects, losses, or inequitable distribution. There are several common forms which interests take in planning:

- A *vested* interest is an advantage already possessed. Vested interests want to preserve and increase those advantages.
- The *public* interest is whatever is to the advantage or benefit of the society as a whole. Some planners apply this only to the collective aggregate economy without reference to who gets what. Others define it as the greatest good for the greatest number of individuals.
- *Private* and *special* interests favor a particular individual, organization, or group.
- *Self* interest is "regard for one's own advantage or profit." Predators do so without regard to consequences for anyone else.
- *Enlightened* self-interest seeks to promote one's actual long run self-interest via something which also benefits others.
- *Disinterest* is not being influenced at all by self-interest. One form of this is *altruism*. Another is *detachment*. Supreme Court justices are appointed for life with high "perks," in

hopes that they will have nothing to gain or lose personally from their decisions.

There are *perceived* interests (what you think is best for you) and *actual* interests (what is really best for you). I think it is in my interest to eat steaks and fries. My doctor says it is actually in my interest to eat more beans and rice.

Traditional science-, engineering-, and economics-oriented planners rely on elite expertise to determine objectively what is in the actual best interests of their targets, whether the latter like it or not: "I'm only doing this for your own good." Critics say that such determinations are not objective but perceived, biased by their various beliefs and interests.

Humanistic planning approaches such as advocacy, transactional, learning-adjustment, disjointed incremental, and political planning stress self-determination based on the perceived interests of those to be affected, regardless of how wise or foolish those wishes may be. "Actual" best interests are not studied.

Some hit a middle ground in which the planner gives "technical assistance" to help actors move their perceptions closer to actual enlightened self-interest.

As planners, we are wise always to discover both actual and perceived interests, how they may affect the project, and how the tension between them can be handled.

Values and Interests Entwined

Values and interests are so closely entwined as to be virtually inseparable when it comes to making planning choices. Values define *what* interests are more important. Graduate education or owning a home? Salary or intrinsic job satisfaction? Endangered species or logging exports? Medical care or public education?

Values guide decisions on whose interests take preference. Investors or workers? Children or senior citizens? Suburban commuters or inner-city bus riders?

In the opposite direction, interests influence value choices: consciously, unwittingly, or perhaps ambiguously. Saul Alinsky (1972, pp. 42-43) put it bluntly:

The purpose of the Haves is to keep what they have. There-fore, the haves want to maintain the status quo and the Have-Nots to change it. The Haves develop their own morality to justify . . . means employed to maintain the status quo; . . . any effective means of changing the status quo are usually illegal and/or unethical in the eyes of the establishment. Have-Nots, from the beginning of time, have been compelled to appeal to 'a law higher than man-made law.' Then when the Have-Nots achieve success and become the Haves, they are in the position of trying to keep what they have and their morality shifts with their change of location in the power pattern. Eight months after securing independence, the Indian national Congress out-lawed passive resistance and made it a crime.

Much of the time, the interplay between interests and values is obvious. Would you expect anyone to hire a trial lawyer who did *not* selectively slant everything possible, including values, toward the client's interest? You have to look for it more carefully when it is cloaked in hypocrisy—or when good folk are deceiving them-selves.

Knowing value-interests, both yours and others', and where they come from does not tell you whether they are right or wrong, or what to do with them. But knowing "where it's at" enables you to play with the full deck. You can make better choices, develop wiser strategies, and protect yourself better. For example, your chance of success may be highest when you can come up with a proposal in which appeals to actors' altruistic values "coincide" with enlight-ened self-interest: "doing well by doing good." After forty years of squelching every major health plan, the physician lobby in 1965 went along to Medicare because (1) it was needed by deserving, hurting older people, and (2) it increased the doctors' incomes.

Competing Value-Interests

What is "welfare" for some groups may be "illfare" for oth-ers.

—*Richard Titmuss*

You can't maximize all interests at once. In any plan there will be winners and losers, either in absolute terms or at least relative to each other's outcomes. My Nebraska program also serves western Iowa. In a recent class, two-thirds of my students paid the on-campus tuition rates of $75 per credit for residents, while the Iowans paid the nonresident rate of $175. Off-campus courses at the downtown continuing education center charge all students $85 regardless of residence. What is the effect of moving my three-credit class of thirty students downtown?

- Twenty students will pay more; ten will pay less. The majority are worse off. Should we stay on campus where the majority are better off?
- The ten will save a total of $2,700 at the cost of $600 to the others, resulting in a net saving of $2,100 for the class as a whole. Should we go downtown where the best aggregate pay-off is?
- The $270 savings for each of the ten are significant since most of them are lower- to middle-income. Should the others agree to go downtown because the benefit to their friends outweighs the affordable $2 per week it costs them?

How do you decide? That is a key planning problem! There is no one perfect solution. This much is clear: you *will* make a decision reflecting some value-interest—explicit or implicit.

It is rare not to have conflicts among values. Even an individual has conflicting internal values. I asked a friend why he was depressed. "Last night I had an argument with myself—and I lost."

The most common source of value conflicts is genuine conflict of interest. In our simple case above, each choice favors some interests at the expense of others.

Another is honest value differences. One group seeks to outlaw pornographic movies and books. Another group defends First Amendment freedom of speech and press. Both sides affirm the undesirability of smut and the desirability of civil liberty, but differ on their relative importance. One says that our freedom is so precious that we must endure its porno cost. The other says that porn is so destructive that it justifies a reduction of liberty through censorship. Who is right? Depends on your value premises.

A related source of value conflicts is the tension between *substantive* values which relate to *ends* of a plan (a generous supply of electricity, a secure old age, healthy babies), and *procedural values* which relate to *means* (nuclear power, mandatory withholding for pensions, free universal obstetric and pediatric care).

Finally we encounter a cluster of inconsistencies which cloud the picture. "Will the real Mr. Value please stand up?" An old favorite is the "us/them" *double standards*.

When I was a national church social action leader, I frequently encountered two opposite types of double standard. *Fifty-mile liberals* espoused civil rights in Mississippi, Washington, and South Africa–all more than fifty miles away–but resisted integration of their own Massachusetts neighborhoods. Robert Pinker (1979, p. 3) calls this "the law of telescopic philanthropy . . . that the further away the object of our compassion lies, the more intense will be the feelings of concern and obligation which it evokes." *Caring conservatives*, on the other hand, were generous and compassionate toward people they knew personally while opposing social programs which extended the same treatment to people they did not know.

Compartmentalization muddies the waters. The same person who is genuinely kind and caring in private life may have a cynical value system at work. This is not uncommon, for instance, in competitive business, law, politics, and the military.

Closely akin is the discrepancy between values as *professed* and as *practiced:* "I can't hear what you are saying because what you are doing is speaking so loud." This version is common in such "noble" settings as universities, health services, and churches.

Transcendent and Subordinate Value-Interests

An early scan may reduce the number of value-interests you need to deal with by eliminating those which are simply unacceptable to you as the planner. (However, if they have powerful advocates, you may want to note them for strategic purposes.)

Rank the remaining, legitimate value-interests on their relative importance. You can do it from a right-brained perspective, identifying top overall values, and then fitting in other values as best you can. A friend, Sheldon Rahn, told me a story about his father-in-law, who had been an official of the Federal Council of Churches in the 1920s, supported the labor movement, which heavily represented a different religious and class group from his constituency. Accused of disloyalty and of naively believing that aggressive and sometimes violent unions were more ethical and less self-interested than owners, he reportedly replied, "They are equally self-interested. But God's will coincides *temporarily* with whoever is on the short end of the stick."

If you want to be systematic, you can rank values by the process of paired comparisons. If A takes predecence over B, and B over C, then A is also over C and anything that C is over. For example, I had a student who asserted that nonviolence was at or near the top of her value hierarchy. We probed further, and to our intuitive surprise, it wasn't. She wanted to "get ahead." Would she ever consider violence in the process? No! Well, would she engage in violence to protect her young son? Yes! Would she support her son's fighting in a war, in which he will be violent and risk violent harm? Yes, but only to defend his country in time of peril, but not to pursue geopolitical interests. This produced a neat hierarchy of values:

1. National survival.
2. Her child's welfare.
3. Nonviolence.
4. Desire for gain.

Obviously, when one value is made transcendent, the subordinate ones become *relative*. Whether and how they apply depend on the situation. Some may be mutually supportive with the transcendent ones and each other. Apply them so that they reinforce each other. Some may be parallel, neither supporting nor conflicting. Apply them as resources permit. Reject or compromise, as necessary, conflicting subordinate value-interests.

A good planner will try to find ways to reconcile conflicting value-interests where possible. In the downtown tuition example, there is a possible solution where nobody loses: *compensation*. If each of the ten gainers reimburse two of the other students their $30 losses, the gainers are still $210 ahead ($270 - $60), and there are no losers.

Sometimes compensation is not possible or not satisfactory to the losers. Choosing one interest at the expense of the other may be a necessary evil. However, a good planner looks creatively for win choices which eliminate or reduce value and interest conflicts. In the above case, such a solution might be interstate reciprocity, by which Iowa and Nebraska each charge in-state tuition to residents of the other state. Then we can hold the class on campus at the $75 rate for all. And there is a bonus for "bystanders": all Nebraskans would have a wider choice of affordable colleges.

Probably one of the most successful efforts at win planning solutions was TVA planner David Lilienthal's dialogues with the local people, which led to accomplishing his interests (economic development and flood control) and serving theirs (maintaining old values, beauty, and fishing). In writing this up, Phillip Selznick (1949) coined a new term: co-opt, or "choose together." (Do not confuse the real thing with a corrupted version in which one party takes over a movement through manipulation and subterfuge–the opposite of choosing together.)

BELIEFS AND SLANTS

Whatever is, is right. But purblind man
Sees but a part o' the chain, the nearest links;
His eyes not carrying to that equal beam,
That poises all above.

—John Dryden

A *belief* is "an acceptance of something as true, real." I believe the earth is round. I believe my wife loves me.

A *slant* is "a mental leaning or tendency; bias; point of view." Beliefs both affect slants and are affected by them. Beliefs, influenced by slants, determine planning choices.

Before-the-Fact Beliefs

A priori beliefs "furnish the basis of experience" through *preconceptions about reality,* I have three pairs of sunglasses, tinted green, blue-gray, and yellow. The yellow pair is great on gloomy days. It makes them look sunny. The green pair is nice for driving. It cuts the glare without diminishing the color of the trees and grass.

The blue-gray pair deepens the color of ocean and sky on a too-bright beach day. But they have other effects. The blue-gray dulls the greenery and makes an ordinary day look like the Bronx in winter. The green destroys the azure of tropical sky and sea. The yellow squelches beautiful color contrasts. Perhaps I should get a fourth pair. They say rose-colored glasses make *everything* look good!

A priori beliefs color the reality you see. Three respectable persons observe the same seven-year-old ghetto child reading poorly. One sees "genetic inferiority." Another sees a "culture of poverty." The third sees "institutionalized racism." What are their "facts"? Reality after it has been selectively *filtered* through their tinted sunglasses.

After-the-Fact Belief: Direct Experience

Another kind of belief is *a posteriori*, "based upon actual observation or upon experimental data."

In daily practice, much of our operating belief is *projected from our direct experience*. Shelley hopefully asks the West Wind, "If winter comes, can spring be far behind?" Based on previous personal experience, I agree (although last February I began to wonder!). This is a primary and often highly reliable source of common sense and intuitive insight. "No one should leave home without it." Still, if we don't take a critical look at it, it can lead us astray. Can we count on Shelley's spring if we are stationed on the Ross Ice Shelf in Antarctica?

The limits on generalization from individual direct experience are dramatized by John Saxe in "The Blind Men and the Elephant":

> It was six men from Indostan
> To learning much inclined,
> Who went to see the Elephant
> (Though all of them were blind).
> That each by observation
> Might satisfy his mind.

One man feels its leg and concludes an elephant is like a tree; another feels its tail and says it is like a rope; a third feels its trunk and describes it is like a snake; etc. Each is partly right but wrong about the big picture.

We can guard against overly narrow projections of "fact" by pooling experiences. We can test our own against those of others. We expand our outreach to include empirical data, descriptive and anecdotal accounts, case studies, journalism, television news, biographies, documentaries, and historical accounts. We may extend our insight further through good poetry, literature, art, and drama.

Widening the base and evaluating the sources give us a better chance to fill gaps and sort out the "real" facts. Still, we must be alert to pluralistic pitfalls. Six heads may be better than one at describing an elephant, but how accurate would a composite of Saxe's six learned men be? Nor can we be sure that mixing colors will create a rainbow. Allan Sherman, a popular comedian in the 1950s, recalled the rinse water for his school paint brushes, and observed, "A committee is a place where everyone puts in a different color and it comes out gray."

After-the-Fact Beliefs: Scientific Data

Most professional planners are more comfortable basing their beliefs about reality on "objective" facts, that is, systematically collected and processed *scientific* and *technical* data. Based on statistical correlations in national epidemiological studies, I believe that cigarettes are associated with respiratory problems and cause half a million premature deaths each year. (Not everyone agrees. "I have already made up my mind. Don't confuse me with the facts.")

This too has its limits. However extensive and well-analyzed, gaps and distortions remain. We never have all the relevant information. Not all of it is available, and from what is, we necessarily slant our selection according to what we believe to be most important, our degree of comfort with the information, and how much we can afford to do.

Not even the best scientific discipline can prevent selectivity. The most glaring one is that science is restricted to what can be measured and quantified. This automatically "de-selects" everything else. This is a problem if the planner is a "One Note Charlie" who excludes all elements that do not fit his research method.

Even within its area of competence, science must be selective.

Nuclear physicist Heisenberg (1958) warned that "What we observe is not nature itself but nature exposed to our method of questioning." Fellow physicist Franz Capra (1984, pp. 126-127) agrees:

> The observer decides how he is going to set up the measurement and this arrangement will determine, to some extent, the properties of the observed object. If the experimental arrangement is modified, the properties of the observed object will change in turn. . . . When observing a subatomic particle, one may choose to measure—among other qualities—the particle's position and its momentum. These two quantities can never be measured simultaneously with precision. We can either obtain a precise knowledge about the particle's position and remain completely ignorant about its momentum or vice versa; or we can have a rough and imprecise knowledge about both qualities.

Another factor is operating too. "The scientist cannot play the role of a detached objective observer, but becomes involved in the world he observes to the extent that *he influences the properties of the observed objects*" (Capra, 1984, p. 127. Italics supplied).

If all this is true for rigorous "hard" scientists, how much more for social and behavioral scientists, applied professionals, and politicians, not to mention us ordinary folk?

Other Slants

We have seen how a priori beliefs and previous experience select and color what we see. To this we can add emotional factors. A news item on teen smoking reported, "One 17-year-old senior at West Henderson High School explained, 'I know it's bad for me, but I'm young still and I think teenagers don't really worry about it'" (Hendersonville, NC, *Times-News*, February 17, 1994).

Wishful thinking biases one toward unrealistic expectations. "If wishes were horses then beggars would ride." Less extreme in the optimistic direction is a generally happy, upbeat disposition. Slanting the other way are depression, alienation, and hostility.

Another set of slants develops from errors in reasoning, which we will discuss in the chapter on rationality.

These factors not only affect our interpretation of what we see, but also are selective on whether we see it at all. For example, every day, that high-school senior and my wife, a respiratory therapist, both encounter older adults with overt symptoms of emphysema and other smoking-related disorders. My wife sees them. The student doesn't.

Hermeneutics

Gerald Kennedy (1943) said, "Nothing changes more constantly than the past; for the past that influences our lives does not consist of what actually happened but of what men believed happened." The "reality" that influences our planning is not what is but what we believe it to be.

A useful tool in dealing with slants is *hermeneutics*, "the science of interpretation" or as Herbert Kohl (1992) prefers, "the *art and craft* of interpretation (italics supplied)." Hermeneutics is not part of the planning tradition. It emerged from the fields of art, literature, history, and Biblical scholarship, where scholars make their reputations by finding the "real" meanings in Shakespeare, Genesis, or Van Gogh. The outstanding thinker on this subject is Hans Georg Gadamer (1975).

Hermeneutics seeks to correct "the Enlightenment error," the delusion of objectivity, that one can know truth through pure reason that transcends individual bias or our cumulative cultural heritage. However, this error is still dominant in many areas of science, technology, social research, economics, cost benefit analysis, and traditional comprehensive rational planning, but it is fraying at the edges. Science has departed from this detached objective stance on its largest (cosmos) and smallest (subnuclear) frontiers and in "organism biology." So have several newer planning models.

Hermeneutics also seeks to avoid the opposite error of giving up on trying to generalize at all. Classical empiricists such as George Berkeley (1710) and David Hume (1748) said that the only true knowledge was firsthand direct experience, and you cannot generalize reliably about the world from your limited subjective perceptions. Relativism says that you cannot generalize because "it all depends," varying with the individual, time, and circumstances. Existentialism carried it to its logical extreme. Since there was no ultimate purpose or direction, there was nothing toward which to generalize.

Understanding is always *codetermined* by the subject (text, policy, circumstances, conditions) and the *vantage point* of the interpreter. You cannot start with a *tabula rasa* because no slate is blank. Even science, which was intended to achieve detached objectiveness, proved to be, itself, a finite particular vantage point.

Every interpreter, looking from a particular vantage point, will miss or ignore some of what is there, and read into it some things which are not there. The objective is not to become free from prejudgments, for that is impossible. Says Gadamer (1975, p. 239), "the really critical question of hermeneutics is to separate true prejudices by which we *understand* from the *false* ones by which we *misunderstand*." In planning, become as fully aware as you reasonably can of VIBES slants, both yours and those of other key actors. What are they? What are their sources? How will you treat them?

The traditional homiletics' three-part analysis of a biblical text may be a useful model in carrying this out:

- *Exegesis*. Start specific. Where did it come from? What did it mean in its original context?
- *Exposition*. Generalize from it. What are its broader implications which transcend the original setting?
- *Application*. Return to specifics. What does it mean to us here and now? How does it affect our decisions and courses of action in *this* specific plan?

As a simple *aide memoir*, keep a checklist of reference points that regularly influence the VIBES slants of people, such as:

- Sociocultural background.
- Demographic identification: gender, ethnicity, generation.
- Relationship networks: family, friends, neighbors, fellow workers.
- Role models: mentors, parents, successful public figures.
- Sources of ego-affirmation: peers, family, higher status groups.
- Occupational and professional socialization.

- Information sources: their accuracy, completeness, slants, gaps.
- Personal vested interests: career, financial, social, ego.

The Bottom Line: Use a Multiple Approach

Good planning draws upon all three sources of belief: projected experience, systematic empirical data, and a priori. Indeed, it is probably impossible not to. Each has both merit and limitations. Each slants the reality. For planning purposes, our best shot is to test all three against each other:

- How do "objective" facts compare with our own personal experiences and observations? If they don't gibe, we need to test our information further.
- Does either information conflict with our before-the-facts beliefs about human nature, society, and the world? If so, we must try to figure out why the discrepancies exist and how to reconcile them.

The result is a hybrid* truth, which blends scientific and other evidence with common sense and intuitive truths. We do not blindly accept whatever our leaders or opponents tell us. We test them against our best available truth, imperfect and slanted though it may be. At least we know what we believe about the situation or circumstance and to some extent why we believe it, and we have sufficient humility to "stand corrected" when we encounter new insights or information. "In the land of the blind, the one-eyed man is king."

REFERENCES

Alinsky, S. (1972). *Rules for radicals*. New York: Vintage.
Capra, F. (1984). *The tao of physics*. 2nd ed. New York: Bantam.
Gadamer, H. G. (1975). *Truth & method*. 4th ed. New York: Seabury.
Heisenberg, W. (1958). *Physics and philosophy*. New York. Harper & Row.
Irving, W. (1855). *Wolfert's Rest. Roost and other papers*. New York: G.P. Putnam.

---

*Trivia note: *Hybrid* comes from the Latin word for the offspring of a tame sow and a wild boar–a proper metaphor for hybrid truth?

Kennedy, G. (1943). *Of heroes and hero worship.*
Kohl, H.(1992). *From archetype to zeitgeist.* Boston: Little Brown.
Pinker, R. (1979). *The idea of welfare.* London: Heinemann.
Saxe, J. (1985). In Hall, D. (Ed.), *Oxford book of children's verse in America.*
    Oxford, England: Oxford University Press.
Selznick, P. (1949). *TVA and the grass roots: Democracy on the march.* Berkeley:
    University of California.

Chapter 3

Ethics

In the actions of men the end justifies the means. Let a prince therefore aim at conquering and maintaining the state, and the means will always be judged honorable and praised by everyone, for the vulgar is always taken by appearances, and the issue of the event; and the world consists only of the vulgar, and the few who are not vulgar are isolated.

–Machiavelli
The Prince, 1537

In the last chapter, we looked at the interplay of values, interests, beliefs, and their slants in planning decisions. One more element of VIBES is *ethics,* a product of the others.

ENDS: DISTRIBUTIONAL ETHICS

The end (goal) of any plan is to make somebody better off. Given the real competition of interests, there is unequal distribution of benefits and costs. Someone gains more than, or at the expense of, someone else.

This raises the issue of *distributional* ethics. Does it make a difference:

> . . . whether the gainers were those who had less to begin with or the reverse, where "the rich get richer and the poor get poorer"?
> . . . whether the loss is planned in advance or an unexpected "spillover"?

... whether compensation is offered and accepted before the fact?

... whether indemnity ("reimbursement for loss") is paid after the fact?

Social philosopher John Rawls (1971) calls for "a proper balance between competing claims." Fine! But what does that mean in practice? There are several alternative ethical principles (and variations within each) which singly or in combinations guide the distributive decision.

Disregarding Distribution

Three positions dismiss distribution as an ethical consideration, in favor of a transcendent value.

Collectivism subordinates the welfare of the parts (individual, groups) to the interest of the whole. This view has strange bedfellows. Stalin's communism and capitalist welfare economics share a standard of *net aggregate gain*; i.e., all benefits minus all losses without reference to who gains and who loses.

Stalin confiscated peasants' lands and forced them into collective farms for the greater good of the *rodina* (motherland). Welfare economics applied the same principle garbed in more sophisticated, mathematical clothing in a 1980s' executive order limiting enforcement of the Occupational Safety and Health Act to situations where increased safety and health was a profitable investment; that is, the gross economic payoffs of preventing death or disability exceeded the cost of the safety measures. In both instances, the effect on specific individuals was not at issue.

A different perspective makes *property rights* transcendent. This automatically affirms the existing status quo of distribution, whatever it is and however it may have been arrived at. Any gain that can be realized from the use of these assets is exempt from distribution questions.

A third position, *amorality,* comes from a different direction. It dismisses moral standards as irrelevant. In this hierarchy of values, taking care of me and mine and "devil take the hindmost" (Beaumont and Fletcher, 1610) claims precedence over such artificial abstractions as justice, solidarity, or compassion. If you refrain from seeking every possible competitive edge, someone less scrupulous will take advantage of you. I call it the *pyrite* rule*: "Do unto others what they would do unto you if they got the chance."

Strict Libertarian

John Stuart Mill advocated negative freedom (freedom from outside interference):

> The liberty of the individual must be thus far limited; he must not make himself a nuisance to other people. But if he refrains from molesting others in what concerns them, and merely acts according to his own inclinations and judgments in things which concern himself . . . he should be allowed, without molestation to carry his opinions into practice. (Mill, 1859, "On Liberty")

Vilfredo Pareto, a turn-of-the-century economist and sociologist adapted this as an ethical standard, known widely in economics as the "Pareto Improvement" or "Pareto Optimum." The concept is that any action is good if one or more persons gain and no one loses from it.

Equality

The standard language of redistribution implies an *equality* standard: *progressive* redistribution reduces inequality; *regressive* increases it.

When we get down to cases, it is not such a simple criterion. What kind of equality do we mean? Do we mean the *same* or *equivalent?* If we want to treat both children in the family equally at Christmas, do we (1) give *identical* toys to a two-year-old and a ten-year-old; (2) give toys of *equal dollar* value, or (3) give toys that provide *equal pleasure?*

Strictly defined, "equal" is "the *same* quantity, size, number, value, degree, or intensity; having the *same* rights, privileges, abil-

---

*Iron disulfide, commonly known as "fool's gold."

ity, or rank." However, this does not allow for variations in circumstances and preferences, as in the case of the two children at Christmas.

We can solve this problem by broadening it to mean *equivalent*, "equal in value, quantity, force, power, effect, excellence, or meaning." The difference between "same" and "equivalent" can be significant.

In the 1965 Civil Rights Law, "equal pay" referred narrowly to the *same* pay for the *same* work within the *same* company. This ignored widespread salary discrepancies between jobs predominantly held by males and those primarily occupied by females. A proposed alternative, "comparable worth" redefines "equal" as "equivalent": equal pay for different work of *equal value* (literally "equi-valent"), using some common denominator.

To compare, we must have a common denominator for value. A good measure would be *utility*, "the power to satisfy the needs or wants of a person"; that is, how much pleasure or satisfaction it provides our third toy option. (It worked with my children at Christmas.)

In dealing with most adults, this isn't as easy. Try to define a unit of satisfaction that everyone agrees with! Economics has come the closest by reducing it to purchasing power, the ability to *buy* things you want. This enables a system of compensation in money for any loss inflicted or cost incurred. If you total your car in an accident, your insurance will give you that model's current "blue book" value. If the government takes your property for a new expressway, it will pay you its "fair market value."

Is there a dollar equivalency for intangible losses such as a father's death, noise pollution, or breakup of an established neighborhood? The mainstream macro social and physical planning usually says yes, that is fair. Critics say no, but then they face the problem of coming up with a doable substitute.

Do we mean equality of input or outcome? With *input equality*, everyone receives the same or equivalent but may end up unequal (due to how it is used and how much each had to start with). The Declaration of Independence talks about input equality. We are born with an equal right to the pursuit of happiness—but we don't necessarily end up equally happy. The basic Canadian Old Age Security program provides input equality, the same flat-rate pension to every senior citizen. If you had no other income, you would live meagerly. If you were already well off, it could pay for a trip south in the winter.

In *outcome equality*, everyone ends up equal, which may call for unequal inputs to compensate for different starting points. United States Supplemental Security Income (SSI) uses output equality. It sets a minimum income standard, factors in what you already have, and makes up the difference. If the end condition standard is $500 per month, a person with $400 of other income receives $100, while one with nothing receives $500.

Group health insurance is based on outcome equality. It spends more on group members who become ill in order to restore them as much as possible to the same condition as members blessed with "natural" good health.

Another equality variable is "compared to what?" *Vertical equality* compares *all* people: whether anyone is higher or lower, better or worse off than any other. According to the Constitution, Americans have vertical equality in voting and due process.

Horizontal equality makes the comparison only within peer subgroups which have *like circumstances* or *similar needs*. Wage-based Social Security offers horizontal equality (you get the same as everyone else who made the same contributions) but not vertical equality (you get more than low wage workers).

As you deal with the ethical issues of equal distribution, you need to decide what kind of equality relates to your situation.

Equity

Equality sounds pretty good, but is it always fair? A hard working student turns in excellent papers and is rewarded with an A. A party-boy classmate is less conscientious and settles for a "gentleman's C." This is not equal. Should it be? Does the first student deserve a higher reward because he worked harder, or because he produced more?

Distributional *equity* means everyone gets a "fair" share according to what each deserves. (This is one form of horizontal equality: your share is the same as that of others who have comparable merit.)

This part is easy. The tough part is figuring out what "deserving" is—and measuring it. An equity system requires:

- A *common denominator* to measure and compare merit,
- *Agreement* on the specific value assigned to each merit factor,
- Reliable *measures*, honestly and impartially applied, and
- An *implementation* plan in which rewards are actually based on the above.

In business, economic, and human development planning, the standard of "deservingness" for equity purposes is *production*, usually measured by its *economic market value*; that is, how much a buyer is willing to pay for what you "produce." By this standard, a person who hits spheroids with a stick is 150 times as productive as the person who taught him to read and write.

Is this equitable? The market says yes, because he makes money for his employer, which is more than his teacher could claim! Might a better measure be *social contribution*? The problem is that there is no agreement on how to measure it, so we fall back again to what we can measure.

Where output is hard to measure, deservingness for equity is often based on *input* measures as the best available indicator of true worth: the length of training, effort, stress, and level of responsibility that goes into a job. When I was in the government, bachelors degrees started at GS7 or Second Lieutenant, master's degrees at GS9 or First Lieutenant, and earned doctorates at GS11 or Captain. Military promotions were based on the workers' increased capabilities. Civil service grade promotions came with jobs that required higher levels of skill and responsibility.

Procedural Equity

Procedural equity is a three-legged stool. The first leg is the self-responsible individual freedom values of Pareto and Mill. The second is an unequal reward system based on merit. The third leg is a "level playing field" in which everyone has equal access to merit rewards. If all three legs are in place, presumably everyone gets what he or she deserves.

There are two approaches to procedural equity. One is *negative freedom* as defined by Hayek (1960, p. 19): "It is often objected that our concept of liberty is merely negative. This is true in the sense that peace is also a negative concept. . . . It describes the absence of a particular obstacle—coercion by other men."

"As is" equal opportunity is the absence of external barriers to individual competition. Rawls (1971, p. 87) calls this "pure procedural justice." Hiring decisions are based solely on current merit as demonstrated by performance, testing, credentials, and other indicators. They are not concerned about how we got to where we are now. "The great advantage of pure procedural justice is that it is no longer necessary in meeting the demands of justice to keep track of the endless variety of circumstances and the changing relative positions of particular persons" (Rawls, 1971).

This achieves genuine equity to the extent that we have had *past* procedural equity in attaining our current level. When I was a student at Princeton University, which was located within 60 miles of a majority of all Jewish-Americans, it had a reported 10 percent quota for Jews and admitted no women regardless of their ability. Since middle-class women and Jews already had comparable high school records, all they needed for equity was "pure procedural justice." The Princeton my daughter attended after these barriers were removed was half female and perhaps one-third Jewish.

Unfortunately, this is not always the case. By happenstance some of us were born into families that offered many social and educational advantages. Others of us with comparable inherent ability experienced accumulated diswelfares due to what Rawls (1971, p. 54) benignly calls "historical and social fortune." Additional diswelfares are inflicted both by institutionalized race, gender, and class inequities built into our society, and by direct discrimination, abuse, or oppression. While hardships can be overcome, and privileges may be dissipated, pure procedural justice leaves some of us with an unearned advantage or disadvantage. If we did not have prior equal opportunity to arrive at the current competition, procedural equity is a delusion.

To get *full* procedural equity, we need to add *positive freedom*, having the means to actualize the potential offered by negative freedom. Academic freedom is not worth much if you can't read and write. Market freedom is useless if you're broke. This moves procedural equity logically back to the starting point. Accumulated inequities need to be *corrected* by *compensatory* interventions to *equalize* opportunity. This is called *affirmative* action.

These positive provisions can be external, internal, or both. *Internal compensatory development* enables a diswelfared person to achieve parity through education, training, confidence building, and other supports.

External compensatory preference aims to equalize the imbalance between privileged and diswelfared groups in the existing job and training markets. That is, it gives opportunity preferences to underrepresented groups to bring the proportion up to what it would have been if there had been no inequities. A common approach is bonus points. They were originally developed for war veterans who had suffered severe diswelfares in the defense of their country and returned to find the good jobs occupied by those who had not served. Civil service simply added five or ten points to the earned score on entry and promotion exams to offset the stay-at-home advantage.

A variation on this is to develop an as-is-equity pool of qualified candidates and then, within that pool, favor those who belong to the underrepresented groups.

The *quota* system is an interim reservation of a set number or proportion of openings for persons from the diswelfared group until such time as the imbalance no longer exists.

Generally, external compensatory preference is most effective in tandem with internal compensatory development, so that once having achieved full parity, the individual has no need for further compensatory preferences. Ideally, when opportunity has been fully equalized, Rawls' "pure procedural justice" becomes full equity.

Adequacy

Adequacy sets a minimum standard of "enough." The first priority of distribution is to assure an adequate floor for all parties. Above this level other ethical principles may be applied, such as equity or the Pareto optimum.

What is enough? The dictionary give two definitions of adequacy: "barely satisfactory" (subsistence) and "fully sufficient."

Planning for the poor, the less powerful, and "them" (whoever we have no close ties with) tends to apply the bare subsistence definition. Social Security researchers used it when they developed an adequacy standard, the "poverty line," base on the lowest-cost monthly "food basket" that home economists could devise which still met minimum nutritional standards.

Planning that involves middle- and upper-class interests or "us" (whoever we may be) tends to apply a "fully sufficient" definition of adequacy, as in many national health systems, suburban public schools, and interstate highways.

Looking at it from another perspective, adequacy may be defined in absolute or relative terms. *Absolute* calculations are based on specifically defined "objective" standards. For the poverty line it was a food basket. In my local high school, adequate education (signified by a diploma) is defined absolutely as (1) completion of a set of required courses, and (2) passing scores on a battery of competency tests in reading, writing, and math.

Relative adequacy looks at social and psychological factors, such as self-esteem, satisfaction, status, respect, and social integration. It defines adequacy in comparison to the "normal" level of a community, region, or nation. Definitions of income adequacy have tended to fall in the range of 50-75 percent of median income.

Even "absolute" standards are influenced by time, place, culture, the economy, and politics. In my father's day, eighth grade was the standard of adequacy. In my generation it was high school. In today's job market, a good argument can be made that anything less than post-secondary education is inadequate. The official poverty line was set 25 percent below the researchers' standard when it was discovered that two out of every five Americans were below it, a politically unacceptable statistic.

DOES THE END JUSTIFY THE MEANS?

One of the stickiest ethics areas is between ends (substantive) and means (procedural) values.

Ends are about outcomes. In a health care plan, *who* is covered? Only employees and their families? Selected population categories based on demographics, such as age, income, gender, geographic location? All citizens? All legal residents? All persons taken ill within the country, including visitors and illegal immigrants? What is covered? Acute conditions only? Primary and secondary prevention? Chronic care? "Heroic" efforts where there is little chance for recovery?

Procedural values relate to *means, how* things are done. Given an end of universal health services, should they be directly administered as in Britain, or purchased from the private sector by a single public insurance program as in Canada—or neither, because the procedural value of free market enterprise, transcends the also-desirable-but-subordinate substantive value of universal coverage?

Among major procedural areas are:

- The relative priority of liberty: individual property rights, self-determination, academic freedom.
- How decisions get made: free market, collective bargaining, majority rule, consensus, direct exercise of power, technical analysis, elite experts, judicial due process, divine revelation, trial by combat.
- How the end is achieved.

If there are viable ethical means, there is no ends-means conflict. We discard unethical ones and still succeed. If the values on one side have much higher priority, we usually compromise the other. Often, however, there may be uncertainty as to which is transcendent and to what degree. Ultimately the planner must bite the bullet and make ethics choices, preferably with participation or input from stakeholders and maybe with consultation from an ethicist. But first, look for a creative *win-win "third way,"* like Martin Luther King Jr.'s nonviolent civil disobedience, which satisfied his ethical commitment on both ends and means.

Where conflict exists, there are four responses to the knotty ethical dilemmas involved in balancing ends and means. Does the end justify the means? The answers are: yes, maybe, no, and who cares?

Yes

Yes, the end justifies the means when its value transcends the procedural ethics value. Terrorists, whether Palestinian, Irish or anti-abortion, represent a sincere if frightening extreme. It is not only extremists. In my class, nonviolent mothers were unanimous that they would employ any means necessary, even including lethal violence, to protect their children.

In the Iran-Contra Affair, White House officials sworn to uphold the Constitution sold arms to declared enemies, misappropriated public funds for illegal purposes, and lied to Congress. There was no guilt or remorse. They argued that national security ends took precedence over Constitutional means. Acknowledging a series of illegal actions, Oliver North proudly called his criminal indictment "a badge of honor," claimed publicly to have divine sanction, and later ran for the U.S. Senate on this record.

It All Depends

In the Declaration of Independence, our Founding Fathers justified war in defense of their human rights only after exhausting all other methods:

> Prudence, indeed will dictate that governments long established should not be changed for light and transient causes. . . . But when a long train of abuses and usurpations . . . evinces a design to reduce them under Despotism, it is their right, their duty, to throw off such government. Our repeated Petitions have been answered only by repeated injury . . . we have appealed to their native justice and magnanimity, and we have conjured them by the ties of our common kindred to disavow these usurpations. . . . They have been deaf to the voice of justice. We must, therefore, acquiesce in the necessity [to] hold them . . . Enemies in War.

Many planners take a general position that all things being equal, a good end justifies a bad means only when the following conditions apply.

- *The end is important enough* to warrant extraordinary means.
- *There is no available alternative* means which is less harmful or more ethical.
- *The cost does not exceed the benefit.* Will cheating to get high grades cost you more in competence and employability char-

acteristics than it gained in credentials? Will the displacements caused by your urban renewal plan create more social problems than your program solves? Will censoring textbooks do more to damage freedom than it accomplishes in protecting school children?

- *The means do not subvert the end itself.* Can revolutionaries who overthrow an oppressor avoid becoming oppressors to stay in power against their defeated enemies? Can we get the right message across by spanking (hitting) a child for hitting a smaller one? Can we preserve peace by waging war?

No

No, certain standards of behavior are absolute and cannot be violated regardless of the end at issue. No end can justify a wrong means. Classical economists are so committed to the free market process that the inequality and deprivation by-product effect on many fellow humans is an acceptable "cost."

Martin Luther King, Jr. agreed with the Founding Fathers in affirming government law and order. He also agreed that human rights were a higher value that justified resistance to unjust laws and authorities. At this point, he parted company. He insisted that the resistance must be nonviolent and without malice. Why? Because his religious values transcended violence as a means, even in a just cause:

> Violence as a way of achieving racial justice . . . is immoral because it seeks to humiliate the opponent rather than win his understanding; it seeks to annihilate rather than to convert. Violence is immoral because it thrives on hatred rather than love. It destroys community and makes brotherhood impossible. . . . It creates bitterness in the survivors and brutality in the destroyers. (Quoted in an Omaha *World Herald* editorial, July 12, 1989)

Who Cares?

An *amoral* response asks, "What's the Issue?" Says Saul Alinsky:

The *end* is what you want, and the means is how you get it. . . . The man of action views the issue of means and ends in pragmatic and strategic terms. He has no other problem; he thinks only of his actual resources and the possibilities of various choices of action. He asks of ends only whether they are achievable and worth the cost; of means, only whether they will work. (1972, p. 24)

GRAY-AREA ETHICS

When all is said and done, there are few pure choices in real-life situations. Legitimate interests and values are in tension. No absolute resolution appears possible. In addition, the ethical choices are also influenced by each party's perceived facts about circumstances and expected consequences of alternative courses.

You cannot evade moral responsibility by *default* (failure to act). Not to choose is itself a course of action which can be more harmful than an imperfect active course. "The only thing necessary for the triumph of evil is for good men to do nothing" (Edmund Burke). Theologian Reinhold Niebuhr came to this view. Firmly rooted in a Christian pacifism, he opposed all war under any circumstances, including United States entry into World War II even after Pearl Harbor. Later, as the incredible atrocities and suffering at the hands of the Axis Powers came to light, he supported the war effort because even the horrors of war were a lesser evil than the "sin of irresponsibility" in permitting this to continue.

The General Confession in the old Book of Common Prayer recognized the sin of omission: "We have all done those things which we ought not to have done and *we have left undone those things which we ought to have done.*"

Proportionality

A traditional Catholic gray-area principle is *proportionality.* Identify the positives, including side effects, of each available alternative. Do the same for the negatives. This is easy to say, not so easy to do. It includes projecting your best estimate of all probable consequences (*simulation* in game theory) of each alternative. Weigh the good and the bad in each. Pick the one with the best proportion of good to bad. This is a sort of moral cost-benefit analysis.

Niebuhr's variation on this was called "existential ethics." Like proportionality, it recognized that real life choices are limited, that multiple values and interests are in conflict, and that no "pure" right is available. Make the best choice you can determine in that "existent" situation. Add explicit recognition of human fallibility:

- Limited knowledge of current factors and uncertainties in predicting the future. Some call this "bounded rationality."
- Inevitable bias and slant.
- Inevitable self-interest and self-rationalization.

Then act on your imperfect best judgment, boldly but with a humility that is always open to admitting error and making corrective responses. This, suggests Niebuhr, is better than the alternative "sin of irresponsibility." His students summarized this ethic as "sin bravely and pray for forgiveness."

Utilitarian

As propounded by Jeremy Bentham (1789), utilitarianism chooses the course which does the greatest good for the greatest number. Alinsky (1972, p. 33) puts it bluntly: "To me ethics is doing what is best for the most."

A common application is that it is okay to trade off harm to some individuals for the general welfare. This was the rationale of Caiaphas for executing Jesus after both the Roman governor and the religious council had found no capital offense: "If we let him go on like this, everyone will believe him, and then the Romans will come and take away both our place and our nation. You do not realize that it is better for you that one man die for the people than that the whole nation perish" (John 11:48-50). In fairness to his argument, it was a fact that while the Romans tolerated native religions and cultures as long as they posed no threat to the civil order, they brutally put down any sign of insurrection. Indeed, a few decades later, the Romans did just that, razing Jerusalem and plowing it under.

Relative Impact

Set your priorities according to where it makes the most difference. On the French battlefields of World War I, faced with more casualties than they could handle at one time, doctors developed a priority approach which they called *triage*. Patients were divided into three groups: (1) those who would die despite treatment, (2) those who would live anyway even if treatment were delayed, and (3) those where immediate treatment meant the difference between life and death. Priority was given to #3. Variations on triage continue to be a popular gray-area approach in social, economic, and physical planning.

Feasibility

A final possible yardstick in gray-area ethics may be simply *feasibility*. "A bird in the hand is worth two in the bush." When faced with dilemmas of choice, go with what you know can be done. This is exemplified in a Niebuhr prayer, adapted by Alcoholics Anonymous, "God give me the courage to change what can be changed, the serenity to accept what cannot be changed, and the wisdom to know the difference."

WHAT IS NOT ETHICS

Ethics is often confused with several other normative standards. While they often coincide or are compatible, they should not be mistaken for ethical decisions.

Obviously, this includes *legality*. As Alinsky (1972, p. 42) observed, "The Haves usually establish laws and judges devoted to maintaining the status quo."

This brings us to the second one, religious beliefs. Although my own ethics are religiously based, I have to admit that religion has historically supported some questionable ethics. It is frequently tied to "tribal" self-interest, "us" vs "them." In the 1991 Gulf War, the presidents of both Iraq and the United States asserted that they were guided and supported by God. Could they both be right? (Were either?) In the Inquisition, Jihads, Crusades, and "ethnic cleansing," persecution, abuse, and murder have claimed divine sanction. Religion can be a vessel for special interests, as in the divine right of kings, the Protestant Ethic and capitalism, and a more recent "religious right" movement which promoted political policies advantageous to financial vested interests in the name of Christ who himself taught, "Do not lay up for yourselves treasures on earth."

Democratic process is a cherished norm and a protection against many injustices. But not always. Slavery was permitted by the Constitution as a result of a democratic compromise. Jim Crow segregation was initiated and maintained by majority decision until overthrown by a nondemocratic judicial interpretation of the Fourteenth Amendment in 1954.

Traditional morality is neatly summarized in the twelve Boy Scout laws (trustworthy, loyal, helpful, friendly, courteous, kind, obedient, cheerful, thrifty, brave, clean, and reverent). This overlaps considerably with ethical decisions–but not automatically. Adolph Eichmann was obedient. Thrift has been the rationale for cutting human services such as public education, health care, and aid to poor children. Brave men can be macho bullies. Finally, "loyal" may require adopting an amoral ethical position, as in Stephen Decatur's toast, given at Norfolk, Virginia in 1816: "Our country! In her intercourse with foreign nations may she always be in the right– but our country, right or wrong."

BACK TO VIBES

In summary, there are many ethical dilemmas to resolve in planning. Due to the fallibility described throughout the discussion of VIBES, there is no simple formula or conclusion that can be applied by rote. We have looked at many approaches. The planners ultimately must make their specific decisions in each plan, hopefully guided by self-aware global values, interests, beliefs, ethics, and slants. Perhaps we come full circle and say for all VIBES:

- They are there, whether you recognize them or not, so it is better to identify and clarify them.
- You cannot get away from them, for default simply gives your proxy to someone else who may not do it as well or may be

promoting contrary interests, so it is better to take some initiative and control.
- Determine what your guiding VIBES will be for the plan. Know what your priority rankings are.
- Blended with as much objective information and insight as possible, figure out how they apply to specific situations.
- Develop compatible goals, objectives, strategies, and tactics.

In simple planning for limited objectives, much of this may be accomplished by a rough scan and brief contemplation. As plans increase in scope, longitude, complexity, and importance, the amount of attention to VIBES increases substantially.

REFERENCES

Alinsky, S. (1972). *Rules for radicals*, New York: Vintage.

Beaumont, F. and Fletcher, J. (1610). *Philaster, Act V.* In *Bartlett's Familiar Quotations,* 13th ed., p. 228.

Bentham, J. (1789-1970). *An introduction to the principles of morals and legislation.* London: Althone Press. In Columbia College Staff, *Introduction to Contemporary Civilization in the West,* Vol. II, Chapter 3, Columbia University Press, 1946, p. 817.

Burke, E. In Sedden, G. (Ed.) (1976). *The Great Quotations.* New York: Podent Books.

Hayek, F. von. (1960). *The constitution of liberty.* London: Routledge & Kegan Paul.

Mill, J.S. (1859). "On liberty." In Columbia College staff, *Introduction to Contemporary Civilization in the West,* Vol. II, Chapter 3, Columbia University Press, 1946, p. 817.

Rawls, J. (1971). *A theory of justice.* Cambridge: Harvard University Press.

Chapter 4

Everybody's Got a System

Our little systems have their day;
They have their day and cease to be.

—Tennyson
"In Memoriam," (1850)

I must Create a System or be enslav'd by another man's.

—William Blake
Jerusalem, 1811

The world as we see it is filtered through our systems model. A *system* is "a set of component parts interacting with each other within a larger whole." A *systems theory* is a model of how everything fits together. To reduce complex reality to a consistent, manageable framework, any systems model must be selective and simplified.

Several different systems models are used in planning. The one chosen affects definition of the problem, general approach, analysis, goals, and courses of action. Each holds a measure of insight and truth "in an earthenware pot." Different models are useful in different situations. To select the best model for a given plan, we need to know the assets and limitations of each.

MECHANISTIC SYSTEMS

Closed Mechanistic Systems: Natural Law

The mechanistic systems model, drawn originally from Isaac Newton's laws of mechanics, is the basis for the traditional scientific method, used in engineering, mathematical, technological, macro economic, and several quantitative social research methods.

- It is a *closed system*, operating on its own without outside interference.
- It is a *structured* system, "a fixed arrangement of component parts."
- There is a natural balancing of forces to create an *equilibrium*.

A simplified illustration of a closed physical system is shown below. Water vapor falls as rain onto land and ocean. Land water flows to the sea (or lakes), from which it evaporates back into the air. The cycle maintains a constant total water supply in equilibrium between the liquid and gaseous states. In the chart below, the arrows show the flow of water molecules:

WATER VAPOR

↑   ↓

rain evap

↓ ↓ ↑

LAND ›SEA

An economic version, postulated by nineteenth-century economist Jean-Baptiste Say, is known as Say's Law—*Supply creates its own demand*. Like the water, total money supply is constant, nothing coming in or going out. It goes around within its closed cycle, maintaining equilibrium between supply (production) and demand (consumption). Producers pay workers to make the goods. The workers spend it on the goods. This returns it to the producers who use it to pay workers to produce more, enabling them to buy more products, etc. In the following chart, the arrows show the flow of money:

PRODUCER ← SUPPLY

↓   ↑

WORKER   › DEMAND

A problem with closed systems is there aren't any. In real life, no system is ever completely self-contained. Everything smaller than the universe is a *subsystem* of something bigger, which we may call "environment" or "larger context." I am a system—which is part of a family—which is part of a community—which is part of a state—which is part of a nation—which is part of the Earth—which is part of the solar system—which is part of the Milky Way, etc. Each system also has *interfaces* (common borders) with other systems (other individuals, groups, businesses, nations, etc.). "Intervening variables" come in, and "spillovers" go out.

The water-cycle system assumes a constant supply of water in liquid and gas form. This is not entirely true. Photosynthesis *eliminates* water (H_2O) molecules, using their atoms to make carbohydrates. Burning of carbohydrate fuels (wood, natural gas, etc.) creates new water. Some water leaves the water-cycle system as it sinks down into groundwater or freezes into the ice cap. Irrigation from wells or global warming puts it back into circulation.

Say's Law assumes a constant money supply. Not so in real life. Credit puts new money into circulation when it is borrowed, and takes it back out later when it is repaid. Putting money in your mattress instead of respending it takes it out of circulation. Foreign trade takes money out of our national supply when imports are bought, and brings it in when exports are sold. Say's Law is reliable to the extent that the system is genuinely closed (an isolationist cash economy) or the ins and outs offset each other.

Semi-Open Mechanistic System: Production Model

The production model is still mechanistic: a finite, orderly world where constants can be analyzed and calculated mathematically, but with a front door added to receive inputs (needed resources) and a loading dock in the rear for outputs (finished products). Feedback affirms its effectiveness and/or identifies production problems. The chart below shows the basic production model and (in parentheses) the human service version:

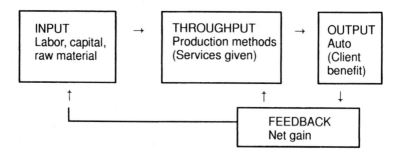

The *economic production model* reduces all inputs and outputs to a single common denominator–money–permitting comparison of alternative courses of action:

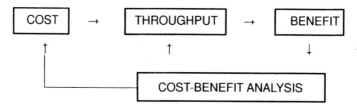

Cost is the dollar value of the input. Benefit is the dollar value of the result. In business, this is revenue from selling the product; in human services, the economic value of desirable changes in the client. Cost-benefit analysis determines the net gain. In business, this is profits; in human services, net contribution to the overall economy.

This model is used to select the course of action with the best payoff. First, is it worth doing at all? Yes, when the dollar value of the benefits is greater than that of costs. Second, among worthwhile choices, which is the best buy? The one with best benefit-to-cost ratio (e.g., a payoff of $3 per $1 of cost is better than $2 per $1).

Misapplications are a frequent pitfall of this model, especially in relation to human services. *Pseudoefficiency* calculates cost per unit of input (such as a course or a counseling hour) instead of cost per unit of output (such as educational growth or social adjustment). The reason is very human. It is easier than trying to measure the intangible outputs, a problem the business version of the model doesn't have because its bottom line really is money.

Another pitfall is *myopia* (nearsightedness). In Japan, the business culture gives priority to long-term gains rather than short-term payoffs. There are cost-benefit methods for estimating this. On the other hand, American businesses and government usually look only at the short term. The reason for this is also very human. What most investors and elected officials care about is this year's profits or next year's election.

Scientific Challenges to Mechanistic Systems

Classical science uses the mechanistic model. When it encounters things that do not fit neatly into the model, especially the qualitative dimensions and dynamic processes of life, it limits its inquiry to what it can measure, and like Aesop's fox, says that data isn't important anyhow. Positivism carried this to its logical extreme, asserting that the out-of-reach grapes do not exist at all.

Newer science rediscovered Heraclitus' flux:

> Relativity eliminated the Newtonian illusion of absolute space and time; quantum theory eliminated the Newtonian dream of controllable measurement process; chaos eliminates the Laplacian fantasy of deterministic predictability. (Gleick, 1987, p. 6)

Adds Crichton (1991, p. 158):

> Mathematicians believed that prediction was just a function of keeping track of things. If you knew enough, you could predict anything. . . . Chaos theory throws it right out the window because in fact there are great categories of phenomena that are inherently unpredictable.

Application to Planning

The mechanistic system model followed engineers, the early planners, into physical planning. In business, engineering efficiency experts applied it as "scientific management" of production, where it mated with the profit system and begat the economic production model.

It offers two key assets, which are also the roots of its limitations. First, it reduces an incredibly complex world to *measurable quantitative data* which can be analyzed by "crunching numbers." The price of this neatness is that there is no place in this system for intangible human elements that cannot be reliably measured.

Its second asset is to make projects or situations manageable step by step. Because the whole structure is fixed with everything in its proper place, it can be broken down into bite-size pieces. You can analyze the parts separately and can add up bits of information. Similarly, you can carry out the plan piece by piece and then put it back together according to the master structure. The whole is the sum of its parts: no more, no less.

The flip side of this is tunnel vision, which lacks perspective on the whole system and misses important external factors.

When is this an appropriate system model for planning? Where the focus is impersonal and material, and the impact of externals is minimal, this simple and easy model is close enough to work very well. As external effects and qualitative considerations increase, it gets in over its head.

In planning a town water system, this model may be efficient and as accurate as you need, but it is inadequate for dealing with the complex interactions of a regional watershed plan.

A single student going to college full time with parental support may be able to treat his or her academic planning as a closed system. How well would that work for a classmate who is a single mother of three, juggling job, family, and studies?

On the personal planning level, I can plan a summer trip from Nebraska to Florida with my computerized automap program, a flat-map system of numbered highways that takes into account mileage and the average speed on two–lane versus four-lane roads. Its shortest route southeast through the Ozarks is indeed the quickest way. However, in winter I must take weather variables into account. The best route may be to detour away from a snowstorm, to take a longer but flatter route to avoid slippery mountain roads, or to head straight south to escape snow and ice sooner. This is beyond the mechanistic automap's capacity.

Even when it is inadequate for the plan as a whole, it doesn't mean I have to throw it out as unhelpful. I start by running all of the automap's alternatives: shortest, quickest, or expressway-preference. Then I tailor-make my own personal plan, using information from all three printouts, and factoring in such things as the weather, my leisure-pressure quotient on this trip, and a "blue highway" see-America interest.

In addition, after a strategic plan has been developed within a broader dynamic perspective, mechanistic may be the way to go for specific subplans. Once a dam is approved and funded, its construction plan may be most effective with a mechanistic engineering system. Project management's mechanistic critical path method has proved its worth in designing implementation of a plan under relatively stable and controllable conditions.

ORGANISM-BASED SOCIAL SYSTEMS

The Systems Theory of the Organism

In the 1920s, Ludwig von Bertalanffy criticized fellow biologists for following Descartes' *deconstructionist* treatment of "the organism as a caloric, chemical-dynamic, cellular, cybernetic animal machine" which can be known by dissecting it into its parts, analyzing them separately, and adding them up. He called for a *gestalt* ("whole") approach to the organism as a complete whole whose properties can not be deduced from simply looking at the parts.

In the late twenties von Bertalanffy wrote:

> Since the fundamental character of the living thing is its organization, the customary investigation of the single parts and processes cannot provide a complete explanation of the vital phenomena. This investigation gives us no information about the coordination of parts and processes. . . . The properties and modes of action of higher levels are not explicable by the summation of the properties and modes of action of their components taken in isolation. If, however, we know the ensemble of the components and the relationships existing between them, then the higher levels are derivable from the components. (1975, pp. 150-153)

In *Jurassic Park,* Crichton (1991) distinguished between consistent, predictable mechanistic systems and organism systems, which fluctuate and change continuously, both internally and in response to the environment:

> Resonant yaw means that even though a missile was only slightly unstable off the pad, it was hopeless. . . . That's the feature of mechanical systems. A little wobble can get worse until the whole system collapses. But those same wobbles are essential to a living system. They mean the system is healthy and responsive.

"Organismic biology" describes a dynamic living system whose characteristics include:

- An *open system*, exchanging matter and energy with the environment. As in the production system, but with more complexity and variability, there is input, throughput, and output.
- *Metabolism*, taking inputs from the environment (food, air) and processing them to meet organism survival needs.
- *Morphogenesis,* changing form through growth, development, and regeneration.
- *System maintenance*, whereby the parts (e.g., organs) contribute to the survival of the whole system, which in turn nourishes the parts.
- *Self-correcting* restoration and maintenance of equilibrium (sweating or shivering to adjust body temperature, generation of new cells to replace dying ones, healing of injuries).

From Organism to Social System

Bertalanffy extended his "systems theory of the organism": "This was the germ of what later became known as *General Systems Theory* (italics supplied). If the term 'organism' is replaced by 'organized entities,' such as social groups, personality, technological devices, etc. this is the program of systems theory" (1975, p. 152). From this, modern *Social Systems Theory* was derived.

Assets of the Social Systems Model

This model more accurately reflects the dynamic reality of individuals, organizations, economies, or societies than a mechanistic fixed "blueprint" perspective. It anticipates movement, flux, change, forces and counterforces, actions and responses. It is open, recognizing two-way traffic between the system and its environment. It routinely takes uncertainty into account. It makes provision for uncontrolled elements, and is alert to its own spillover effects onto others.

In a fixed system, the single best course of action can be discovered by breakdown analysis. In the social systems model, with its dynamic interplay of many factors, there may be more than one way to skin a cat. This encourages the planner to search out a variety of alternative courses, pick the most promising in this specific circumstance, and allow for unexpected contingencies.

If one entry is blocked, find another way. If antibiotics don't work for the flu, try chicken soup.

For instance, my denomination had a goal to integrate women fully into the clergy. They were blocked from regular pastorates by traditional local church identification of "pastor" with "father." Instead of confronting this closed front door, they used an upstairs window. If you can't start at the bottom and work up, why not start at the top and work down? Outstanding female clergy were recruited and promoted to highly visible leadership positions in the state conferences and national headquarters. After a while, female clergy leadership became seen as normal, and slowly but steadily congregations opened up without contention.

Another asset of an organism model is the opportunity for *synergism*, "the simultaneous action of separate agencies which together have greater effect than the sum of their separate individual effects." If your goal is vocational rehabilitation, you may want to cluster a "battery" of mutually reinforcing interventions, such as physical therapy, emotional counseling, and skill training. If you further yoke this with economic development to create jobs, and an education program to persuade employers to hire the handicapped, the effect of the package exceeds the total of what each would have achieved by itself.

Limitations of the Social Systems Model

A social system is *not* an organism. It is more complex. The model is too small. (Counterargument: yes, but all models must be simplified enough to use in a practical way. This reduction is a reasonable compromise.)

Further, the parts are not organs; they are people. They are not totally dependent on the system nor is the system dependent on its parts in a fixed way. They can emigrate out of the system, move around within it, change their system functions. They may pursue separate self-interests at the expense of other parts, as in slavery, crime, and unregulated monopolies.

In an organism, system maintenance is a biological necessity. Production's primary function is survival. This is also the case for some social systems, such as a subsistence economy. For certain other social systems, such as an industry or a social agency, it's the other way around. System maintenance is merely a means to its primary purpose, production.

In broad social planning, maintenance and production are often in tension with each other. For instance environmental protection and occupational safety (system maintenance) clash with maximum economic production.

COMMON PROBLEMS IN APPLYING SYSTEMS MODELS

Limitations of both the mechanistic and the organism systems theories lead to several common (but not inevitable) pitfalls.

The very concept of a "system" is biased toward the collective as more important than individual parts. This is absolute in the mechanistic model and dominant in the organism one. That is not what we profess in our secular and religious faiths:

> That to secure these Rights, Governments are instituted among men, deriving their just powers from the consent of the governed, That when any Form of Government becomes destructive to these ends . . . it is the Right of the People . . . to

institute new Government . . . in such form, as to them shall seem most likely to effect their Safety and Happiness. (Declaration of Independence)

The Sabbath was made for the sake of man, and not man for the Sabbath. (Mark 2:27)

This is why the global level is necessary for planning. That is where we, not the systems model, set our ultimate goals and priorities, determining the balance between the interests of overall systems and those of its individual parts. If we don't, the latter tend to get short shrift.

As a macro planner in a federal program in which 100,000 living, breathing, feeling children were referred to as "zero point one (million)," I had to work at keeping focused on the bottom line: each child.

A frequent systems pitfall is to give a conservative slant to the key concept of equilibrium. It tends to oppose anything which may upset the balance, thereby supporting preservation of the status quo, good or bad. However, this is an ideological overlay, not inherent in systems. An organism system can and does create new, better equilibria. Health authorities encourage persons who have no current disorder to "get into shape," which entails shedding pounds, rearranging what's left, building muscle tone, and increasing aerobic capacity. For some of us this new, healthier equilibrium is a long way from "status quo." Economic development is another change-oriented move to establish a new higher equilibrium for productiveness and living standards.

Systems thinking tempts one to get too complex in planning and analyzing. Most executives, politicians, and ordinary people do not study topics in great depth. However valid it may be, too much of a good thing may confuse or simply turn them off. Is a simpler model sometimes wiser?

Ironically, an opposite pitfall is to use a systems model as a copout in the face of dauntingly complex situations. For instance, the economic production model permits you to reduce everything to a single, measurable element: dollars. Simplification is good. But what have you lost in the process? Does it lead you too far astray?

Finally, there is the temptation to *reify*, "treat an abstract concept as if it were a concrete or material thing." Ignoring the discrepancies between a model and real life, the model itself replaces the reality it was intended to represent. President Hoover's reification of the classical free market economic system model crippled his capacity to cope with (or even recognize) the disastrous effects of the Great Depression.

WORLDVIEWS

A *worldview* (from the German *Weltanschauung*) colors how we see the world. It is an umbrella belief about how people and society actually function. It may be a product of both experience and a priori ideologies. While it may influence our broad values and goals, it has a particular impact on selecting specific objectives and means.

Unitary-Collective

This view sees society (or a large organization) as a collective entity. The whole and its parts are interdependent, with the priority being to optimize the total system, even at the expense of its parts (members). "Ask not what your country can do for you, but what you can do for your country" (J. F. Kennedy). It may use a mechanistic model of society as a watch with internal wheels and cogs, or an organism model of society as a body with a complex of organs.

This worldview supports centralized, comprehensive rational planning by presumably disinterested experts. "Father knows best." We find this in such areas as economic development, military defense, business corporations, community master plans, infrastructure development, and large human service programs.

Plural-Collaborative

The collaborative worldview also sees a society or organization as an integrated social system, but with a key difference. It is pluralistic. The overall system is not an end in itself but a means for enhancing the pluralistic interests of its members, who interact in a mutual give-and-take spirit. There are two versions, according to whether one believes resources are fixed or open.

The *fixed sum* version focuses on *distributive justice*. Competing interests compromise for less than they want in order that everyone may have a fair share of what is available. The ideal, where feasible, is for me to concede to you that which is unimportant to me but high priority to you, and vice versa. "Jack Sprat could eat no fat, his wife could eat no lean, and so betwixt the two of them, they licked the platter clean."

The *open end* version focuses on optimizing each part. Its planning focus is often developmental. The minimum is a Pareto Improvement, whereby someone benefits at no cost to others.

Better are win-win developments. All sides come out ahead. The United Negro College Fund's motto expresses this: "A mind is a terrible thing to waste." Message: a college education benefits the targeted individual, who in turn contributes more to society. Social Security pensions help the aged and free their middle-aged children from former burdens and increase merchants' revenue *and* stabilize economic cycles.

Planning within a collaborative worldview tends toward high participation of targets and actors who work out mutually acceptable outcomes. This has been the style of planning in the federated voluntary service field, through such mechanisms as Jewish Federations, United Ways, and Councils of Churches. Other collaborative worldview applications include Banfield's politicized rational planning (Meyerson and Banfield, 1955), Lindblom's "partisan mutual adjustment" (1968), Friedman's "transactional planning" (1973), and corporations' "TQM" (total quality management).

Plural-Competitive

> One must either be the hammer or the anvil.
>
> *—Peasant proverb*

A third worldview is that we live in a predatory jungle. John Locke (1690) described "man in the state of nature" as free but in constant danger from predatory fellow men. He reluctantly proposed a collaborative social compact that traded freedom for security. His contemporary, Thomas Hobbes (1651), was more pessimistic in his description of a state of nature: "No arts, no letters, no society, and, which is worst of all, continual fear and danger of violent death, and the life of man solitary, poor, nasty, brutish and short." This worldview was carried to its logical extreme by nineteenth-century Social Darwinism, which believed that the world not only *was* predatory but *should* be.

There is no such thing as "the general welfare" as this world turns. There are only competing interests. It's the coyote against the rancher. Coyotes attack calves to eat them. Ranchers shoot the coyotes to save the calves–who are eaten later by humans.

Distribution is unequal, based on power alone. "Him that has, gits." "Fair (fare) is what you get on the bus with." Among those who believe most strongly in this reality are aspiring entrepreneurs on one side, and oppressed people on the other.

Planners with this worldview pay close attention to power resources. Advocacy planning is the logical approach for this worldview. You will go for your interests. I shall go for mine. There will be no voluntary sharing. If we have more power, our interests will gain. If our power is inadequate, we settle for the best we can salvage under the circumstances–and make our first planning priority *empowerment* sufficient to become a player in the next game–or its controller.

Plural-Compartmental

The final worldview does not address systems at all, unitary or pluralistic, predatory or benign. Maybe there is a big picture. Maybe there isn't. Either way, it is out of your reach to do anything about it. What you *can* do is:

> Build a sweet little nest
> Somewhere in the West,
> And let the rest of the world go by.

> *J. Brennan, 1919*

Astute social developers take this worldview when they focus on helping rural third-world villages, which can count on little outside support, to better their lives modestly on their own through self-help "bootstrap" planning. So does much of our personal planning of careers, education, nest eggs, vacations, or retirement. Sure, we take the larger context into consideration, but only as it affects our ability to "brighten the corner where you are."

Can You Mix Worldviews?

In theory, these worldviews are mutually exclusive, yet I find my own worldviews vary. One explanation is that inconsistency is endemic to the human condition. It is more than that, however. We live, existentially, in several different worlds, which vary according to time, place, and circumstances.

In a "lifeboat," the collective worldview is a fact. During World War II, most people shared a collective worldview that "saving the world for democracy," national defense, and liberation of conquered people were collective priorities that transcended comforts, family, even their own lives. In an impoverished economy, the only hope for adequacy is systemwide development.

In the 1950s, macro social workers were taught that "if people of good will meet around a table with the facts, they will make the right decision." This is often true in such planning settings as neighborhood organizations, church projects, collegial curriculum planning, interagency cooperation, and agency program development. The collaborative worldview is accurate when the participants share certain characteristics:

- They have a sense of common identity with each other.
- They start with high consensus on mission, goals, and values, differing mostly on details and "how to's."
- Their vested interests are not significantly threatened by the outcome.
- One or more of them functions as a disinterested process enabler to the others without trying to influence the decisions.

On the other hand, the competitive worldview described what I encountered when I worked in East Harlem, and later in the National Welfare Rights Movement. Our planning had to stress empowerment, coalition, challenge, advocacy, and negotiated settlements. "First you must get their attention. . . ." The collective worldview was a fraud for these people's lives. What the people experienced with landlords, sweatshop employers, public welfare social investigators, the police, and city hall bore no resemblance to a collaborative world. A compartmental view offered band-aid palliatives but didn't change the way the deck was stacked.

The compartmental worldview is real when you are isolated from the mainstream or frustrated by immovable circumstances. As a teacher, I thank God for academic freedom. Regardless of environmental circumstances, I can still help individual students within my own little niche. It also fits the many subareas of our lives that nobody else much cares about.

Where does this leave us? We live in several different "worlds." One is collective. Another is collaborative. Others are competitive. Some are circumscribed. We may therefore act on one worldview in this planning situation, and another within that one. Indeed, one might even use more than one in the same plan. For instance, in community organizing, a collaborative view applies to the subgroup's internal decision making process, while a competitive worldview guides its tactics in the larger community. A corporation's top planning reflects a competitive view of society; its internal organization may be seen as a TQM collaborative world, and operational tasks may be broken down into compartmental subworlds.

REFERENCES

Bertalanffy, L. von. (1975). *Perspectives on general systems theory.* New York: George Braziller.
Crichton, M. (1991). *Jurassic park.* New York: Ballantine.
Friedman, J. (1973). *Retracking America: A theory of transactive planning.* New York: Doubleday.
Gleick, J. (1987). *Chaos: making a new science.* New York: Penguin.
Hobbes, T. (1651). "Leviathan." In *Introduction to Contemporary Civilization in the West,* Vol. 1. Chapter 13 (1946). New York: Columbia University Press, p. 714.
Lindblom, C. (1968). *The policy making process.* Englewood, NJ: Prentice Hall.
Locke, J. (1690). "Of civil government." In *Introduction to Contemporary Civilization in the West,* Vol. 1, Chapter 2 (1946). New York: Columbia University Press, pp. 786-790.
Meyerson, M. and Banfield, E. (1955). *Politics, planning and the public interest.* New York: Free Press, pp. 302-329.

Chapter 5

Be Reasonable

So convenient a thing it is to be a reasonable creature, since it enables one to find or make a reason for everything one has a mind to do.

—Ben Franklin

BEING LOGICAL

Rational planning involves systematic reasoning about data, guided by logic. Some definitions:

- *Reason* is "ability to think, form judgments, draw conclusions, etc."
- *Systematic* is "orderly, methodical."
- *Data* are "things known or assumed from which conclusions may be drawn."
- *Logic* is "the science of correct reasoning; valid induction and deduction."
- *Inference* is "the process of deriving the strict logical consequences of assumed premises."
- *Induction* is "the process of drawing a conclusion from particular facts or individual cases."
- *Deduction* is "inference by reasoning from the general to specifics."

Logic starts with a *premise*, "a statement or assertion that serves as the basis for inferences." Inductive inferences lead from individual instances to general theories and models. An apple falling on his head may not have done the job alone, but Isaac Newton's law of gravity was inferred from many such observations. Sigmund Freud's ego psychology presented a pattern to explain his many patients' behaviors.

Deduction applies an already-established general premise (which may be either an a priori belief or an inductive conclusion from evidence) to specific cases. An example is the 1986 "Pastoral Letter on Catholic Social Teaching and the U.S. Economy" from American bishops, which under the heading, "Principal Themes of the Pasotoral Letter," deduced a succession of progressively more specific inferences from a premise:

13. The person is sacred, the clearest expression of God among us. . .
17. Human rights are the minimum conditions for life in community.
18. Society as a whole, acting through public and private institutions, has the moral responsibility to enhance human dignity and protect human rights.
19. These . . . moral principles . . . give an overview of the moral vision . . . of economic life [which] must be translated into concrete measures. Our pastoral letter spells out some specific applications of Catholic moral principles . . . full employment . . . eradicate poverty . . . halt the loss of family farms . . . relieve the plight of poor nations . . . reaffirm rights of workers, collective bargaining, private property, subsidiarity, and equal opportunity. (National Conference of Catholic Bishops, 1986, pp. xi-xii)

Pitfalls

Planners are susceptible to several common errors in reasoning. One is to generalize from *inaccurate or incomplete data*. An old computer adage is "GIGO: Garbage In, Garbage Out." No matter how faultless its circuitry, a computer can only be as accurate as its inputs (data and program). Logic (and its cousin, mathematics) is like the computer. No matter how perfectly processed, if the input is off-base, so will be its conclusions. This is often exacerbated by careless inferences which exceed the data without a disclaimer, as did Saxe's blind men in describing an elephant.

Another common problem is *confusing an a priori belief with empirical data*. As noted earlier, Herbert Hoover, a brilliant engineer, was unable to plan effectively in the Great Depression because he thought his closed-system free market model was the real world, when in fact it had been undermined by corruption, fraud, speculation, monopolistic practices, wars, and international mercantilism.

A reverse problem is *confusing empirical data with a priori values*. This often takes the form of "what is = what should be." In medicine, some argue that the fact of technological ability to prolong physical life infers an ethical obligation to do so in all cases, without regard to the quality of that physical life. A priori premises which (1) put a supreme value on life, and (2) define it as purely physical survival, support such a course of action. Premises that agree with #1, but define life holistically in relation to body, mind and spirit, support an approach that employs technology to optimize quality of life. A value premise that collective economic interests transcend individual life, would apply the technology only where it produces a net monetary gain. The fact of technology does not by itself support or refute any of these three conclusions.

In making a planning choice, we draw upon both empirical data and a priori beliefs and values at every stage. A good rational planner does this in a conscious, self-disciplined way. Not to do so (irrational planning) can be destructive.

SCIENTIFIC METHOD

Rational analysis is closely associated with *science*, "systematized knowledge of nature and the physical world derived from observation, study, and experimentation." The scientific method tests inferences about fact. Its general procedure:

1. Observe specific cases.
2. Infer theory from experience and observation. (Inductive.)
3. From the theory, develop a hypothesis that predicts future specific cases. (Deductive.)
4. Test the hypothesis by observing those cases. Compare the results observed with those predicted.

5. Revise the theory based on this new information, affirming and extending it where predictions were accurate, revising it where they were inaccurate. (Inductive.)
6. Repeat steps 3 through 5 indefinitely to further refine and extend theory and application.

Experimental Method

Traditional science is based on a closed mechanistic model, which allows for two kinds of variables: (A) *independent* (causes) and (B) *dependent* (effects). The ideal method to test the theory is an experiment. Develop a hypothesis limited to predicting the effect of A on B under controlled, closed-system conditions. Measure B. Add A. Measure B again. Conclusion: any change in B is caused by A. In the "hard" sciences, which deal only with measurable material things, this is relatively possible. You may have done this in high school chemistry class.

Quasi-Experimental Method

Unfortunately, real life is an open system, particularly in its social and behavioral aspects. A third kind of variable, *intervening,* comes in from outside and messes things up. You could call it a weed in the scientific garden. A pure experiment is not possible because we can't put it all into a leakproof box. We have to study it out in the cruel world of uncontrolled intervening variables. Unable to exclude them, science relies on a *quasi* ("in some degree") experiment, in which it tries to hold them constant enough to tell whether A has any effect on B. It goes like this.

- Start with a theory: heavy smoking (A) is a cause of emphysema (B).
- Develop a hypothesis to test it: heavy smokers will have a higher rate of emphysema than nonsmokers.
- Convert it to a *null* ("of no effect") hypothesis: heavy smokers and nonsmokers will have the same rate.
- Select two groups. One group has A (smoking). The other does not have A. To minimize the effect of intervening vari-

ables, make the groups as much alike as possible on everything else, by matching or random selection.

• Measure B (emphysema rate) in both groups. If there is a significantly higher rate of B when A is present, we reject the no-effect null hypothesis, and by elimination support its opposite, that A does increase B.

What is *significant*? Because of the leaky system, unwanted intervening variables might affect B. In any given person, such a variable may be present. With a large number of cases randomly assigned to one or the other group, this should average out to be about the same in both. Statistics of distribution calculate the probability (P) that a given level of difference between A and B will occur by chance. A significant level of difference is one which would occur so seldom that you can assume the effect was not by chance. "P < .05" means you will accept as significant a difference likely to occur by chance less than one time out of twenty. A more rigorous test of significance could be "P < .001" (less than one time in 1,000).

Because weeds are in the garden, quasi-experiments can never absolutely prove a total cause and effect, as the tobacco industry points out. It does not rule out other causes (such as air pollution). It settles for determining whether A is at least one significant contributor to B. For planning, this is usually enough to justify acting on A. With all its limitations, the quasi-experimental method is a useful, widespread tool both in developing a plan and in evaluating its effects afterwards.

Clinical Method

Practitioners such as physicians, therapists, and auto mechanics often use a less rigorous, problem-solving adaptation of the scientific method. While "clinical" is primarily a health term, the same general process is used in *applied* planning in such areas as social policy and administration (numbering below is parallel to the six-step scientific method above):

1. Observe healthy cases (e.g., normal intestinal functioning).
2. Infer standards of "health," typically the absence of a disor-

der or problem. ("Health" is not having a bellyache or diar-
rhea.)
3. Observe the specific case. Compare it to the standard. If there
is a deficiency, develop a set of causal hypotheses, inferred
from experience in previous similar cases. (The patient com-
plains of intestinal problems. The doctor identifies seven
possibilities that fit the symptoms.)
4. Test for the predicted effect of the hypothesis. (For each
hypothesis there is a clinical test. The doctor tests them one at
a time. The first two come out "null" and are rejected. When
the third tests positive, it is accepted, and the doctor looks no
further.)
4A. Repeat the process, this time regarding treatment hypotheses
based on accumulated experience. (There are three alternative treatments for this diagnosed disorder. Based on past
experience, the doctor chooses the most likely and predicts
that it will be effective. It is. If it were not, step 4A would be
repeated with the other alternatives.)
5. If all three are ineffective, it's back to the drawing board with
further step-4 testing of the alternative diagnostic hypotheses, and possibly further step-3 development of hypotheses.
(In the actual case described here, there turned out to be not
one but two separate disorders, each of which was ultimately
treated successfully.)
6. Whereas a researcher would continue to the next step—revising basic theory—the practitioner stops when the specific
problem is solved.

Pitfalls and Assets of Science

Despite the fullest rigor that circumstances permit, all science is
imperfect at best. Not all desirable information is available, and its
quality varies from excellent to poor. Further, the sheer magnitude
of what is available is more than we can handle. Our data collection
and analysis is reduced by the available time, resources, and technical tools we have in hand.

A common pitfall is *pseudo* ("false, pretended") science. This is
easily spotted when practiced by charlatans. Its real danger comes
from scientific and technical professionals who sincerely claim a

level of accuracy and validity beyond the limits of their sources, models, and methods. This is the scientific counterpart to dogmatic religion. In theology, it is the sin of pride; in planning practice, the sorcerer's apprentice syndrome.

For all its flaws, the empirical scientific method offers much insight to planning. Given no possibility of infallible information, it may be the best available. "If a little knowledge is a dangerous thing, where is the man who has so much as to be out of danger?" (Huxley, 1877).

Two simple practices will increase its value and lessen its liabilities. One is to be open about its honest limits so that decision makers and other stakeholders can use their critical judgment too. This will probably increase your influence because others will learn to trust what you do say.

The other is to hedge with multiple sources. These can be as diverse as eyewitness reports, anecdotal accounts, client wishes, personal experience, literature, history, philosophical insights, and professional "lore." This is no absolute protection, but generally, the broader the foundation, the more stable the houses.

NONSCIENTIFIC METHODS

Deductive Logic

Not all rational process is scientific. Greek philosophy and systematic theology are rigorously logical in their rational deduction from clear premises. So is (or should be) the determination of planning goals and ethics.

Heuristic Approach

Heuristics (from a Greek word meaning "to invent, discover") is the trial and error method without the systematic, step-by-step procedure of its scientific-method cousin. Heuristic devices include reasonable working assumptions and intelligent guesses. Act on it, test it out. If it works, great! If not, back to the ol' drawing board and try something else.

On the one hand, its hit-or-miss character can make it disjointed and inefficient. On the other hand, it can be more open-ended, innovative, inventive, and creative than a rigid systematic approach. It uses *educated guesses* which are more than intuition but less than definitive. It may be our best bet when we have to operate without adequate knowledge. It is the primary approach of Lindblom's Successive Limited Choices method which is discussed at length in Chapter 6, and is widely used in certain stages of most other planning models.

The advantages of heuristics can be enhanced and its weaknesses reduced if it is hybridized with the scientific method. In the clinical case example, given on pp. 79-80, the patient had previously visited another doctor whose approach had been purely heuristic. The earlier doctor diagnosed and prescribed in ten minutes. When treatment proved ineffective after a month's time, he was back at square one (and the patient went to the doctor described in the case exapmle). This doctor has also used an heuristic approach, but did so *systematically*. First she made educated guesses about several possible diagnoses that fit the symptoms, not just the most common one. Second, she set about trial-and-error testing of them in an organized way. Third, she went on to treatment choices only after she had verified the diagnosis.

Intuition and Insight

Planning needs are not fully met by the scientific method alone. Many of the most important elements related to social (human) planning are *intangible*, "not easily defined or formulated." We need perspective, how things fit together in the larger picture. We must make decisions based on limited, incomplete evidence, which is often fragmented and inconclusive. This calls for some non-scientific intellectual skills, such as:

- *Sensibility:* "keen intellectual perception; the capacity to respond intelligently and perceptively to intellectual, moral, aesthetic, or psychological events or values."
- *Insight:* "the faculty of seeing into inner character or underlying truth; the sudden grasping of a solution; configurational learning."

- *Intuition* (from the Latin "to look at"): "immediate knowing or learning of something without the conscious use of reasoning."
- *Hunch:* "a strong intuitive impression that something will or can happen. It is a common sense form of predictability" (Steiner, 1979, p. 354).
- *Considered judgment:* "experience-based insight."

In 1904 Max Weber expressed a common attitude toward intuition: "The voluminous talk about intuition does nothing but conceal a lack of perspective toward the object." (Ironically, Weber's own greatness was rooted in extraordinary intuition which he subsequently sought to document.)

A veteran of twenty years in planning and administration was accustomed to sizing up complex situations on several "levels" at once, making strategic decisions, and elaborating a detailed course of action quickly. After he moved to academia, his department chair's annual evaluation described him as "off the wall" because he would come in "over there" when the group was discussing "over here." The new professor argued that it was in fact merely faster-than-average traditional rational analysis: "In every case when asked, didn't I give you a logical step by step progression from 'here' (A) to 'there' (G) through steps B, C, D, E, and F?" The chair admitted this was so.

In fact, he did make intuitive jumps—yet he could still "reconstruct" the logical progression without hesitation. He says this is because his "intuition" is in fact *subconscious* rational analysis. Perhaps he's right. We learn concepts and apply them self-consciously, adapting them to a wide variety of different cases. Gradually we assimilate all of this into our own customized "memory files," called "crystallized intelligence," and perform the process "intuitively." (It is prudent to check the soundness of our intuition by periodically reconstructing it in rational analytic format.)

Another common intuitive process seems to be "right-brained," with holistic flashes of insight. Many creative artists will say so. A friend calls it "a glimpse." My wife calls it "visualizing."

Whatever its nature, great scientists such as Newton and Einstein had it. So do most successful administrators and professionals.

They use it as input in their analysis and planning, testing it against other data and thought processes.

> There is a curious natural law in business that places a premium on managerial imagination–The Bigger the Problem, the Fewer the Facts. This law manifests itself in the necessary paradox of "scientific foreman and intuitive president." Many problems at the supervisor's level can be quantified, analyzed, and optimized down to the last few percent. . . . But most problems at the president's level involve such intangibles that any decision at all takes courage. . . . Thus, this simple law places increasing emphasis on the art of sensing essentials early, of drawing inferences from barely sufficient information. For example, a major decision, by the time it is supported by a solid factual basis, in all likelihood should have been made several years ago. (Mills, 1959, p. 1)

A Note to Intuitive Persons in Anti-Intuitive Situations

Intuition is put down in some circles, usually for doctrinaire reasons. Use it anyway. It is an invaluable planning tool.

If you do, be "bilingual," translating your insights into the language of your audience. An artist has his mind's picture, which he translates into pigments on a canvas. A skilled intuitive thinker copies her mind's picture with rationalistic pigments onto a "left-brained" canvas.

If you want to bring others along with you, "start where the client is." The professor cited earlier still thinks the same way but no longer comes in "over there." His insight and vision guide a patient, enabling process through which he helps his colleagues to find their own way at their own pace. It takes much more time and energy, but at the end of the process they "own" it themselves and are far more committed to carrying it out. He observes that "educator" comes from the Latin root *educere* which means "to lead or draw out."

A comparable bilingual approach can be used by a rational analyst in "right brained" circles. It works best, in both directions, if you yourself have developed both kinds of thinking.

BOUNDED AND NONBOUNDED RATIONALITY

The concept of bounded and nonbounded rationality was developed originally by Herbert Simon in 1957. He made a useful distinction between the two.

Bounded Rationality

Bounded means "restrained or confined." Bounded rationality proceeds logically from *prescribed* assumptions about what is desirable and/or feasible. One boundary is your planning area: subject, geographic area, for whom?

Another is "given" constraints. Create an adequate water supply for the city–without disturbing endangered species or scenic rivers. Plan your individual course of study–within the boundaries of degree requirements. This includes apparent limitations on what realistically can and cannot be done within available resources, time, technical capabilities, and political support. Upgrade the rural highway system–within a $50,000,000 state appropriation.

A less obvious boundary is ways of thinking, as already discussed in relation to VIBES, systems, and the scientific method. Positivists bound their planning to what is material and measurable. Technicians may narrow the limits further to include only what they know how to process. Many planners are bounded by vested interests and ideology: develop a national health care plan–which is commercially profitable and does not require new taxes.

Nonbounded Rationality

O beautiful for patriot dream that sees beyond the years
Thine alabaster cities gleam, undimmed by human tears.

–Katharine Lee Bates
"America, the Beautiful"

Nonbounded rationality is not limited in advance by presumed constraints. This can be written off as utopian fantasy. Some time ago, a nonbounded planning branch was set up at the National Institute of Mental Health. Mainline staffers, whose prevailing focus was on treatment of mental *illnesses*, ridiculed the group as "space cadets." That's why NIMH leadership created the branch: as an antidote to such bounded thinking. Its mission was to develop a holistic perspective on mental health, including its interface with such "outside" elements as racism, sexism, poverty, pollution, and urban crowding.

Nonbounded thinking is essential to good strategic planning. It contributes to better goals and raised sights. Robert Kennedy put it this way: "Some men see things as they are and say, 'why?' I dream things that never were and say, 'why not?'"

It provides a beacon that helps us to stay on course. As the winds and waves toss our boat continuously off course, we still know where we are aiming, so that we can make navigational adjustments. Without this, boats and plans may drift far from their original destinations. I found this especially true as a federal planner. Original good intentions were *always* compromised and watered down by the time they had run the gamut of legislative and political realities, and were implemented by less-than-perfect agencies. Perhaps the most classic case of this was the metamorphosis of the Vietnam War over a twenty-year period.

A certain amount of nonbounded creativity is desirable in selecting and carrying out feasible means. It can't be done? Are you sure? As my old literature professor would say, "Let's walk around it again."

A modest example of this was the need to recruit and retain high-quality minority faculty in a program preparing professionals to serve multicultural clienteles. In a prairie university with below-average salaries, this seemed an unachievable goal. Then a nonbounded thinker said, instead of recruiting PhDs, why not grow our own? They recruited outstanding minority master's-level practitioners with local roots to become "faculty interns," with a full salary, tuition, and released time for doctoral study, plus a tenure-track position upon successful completion. End result: over time, goal fully achieved.

The difficult we do immediately.
The impossible takes a little longer.

—*Army Air Corps, World War II*

REDUCTION

Reduction is necessary in all but the simplest planning and decision making. The complexity of even a small system is beyond our ability to encompass it. One way or another, we have to reduce it to what we can realistically handle and afford.

Exclude Complicating Factors

One way is to limit the number of elements considered to a few key ones. For better and for worse, some of the criteria for omitting elements include:

- *Marginality.* They would not make enough difference to affect the outcome.
- *Capability.* You can't do anything about them anyway.
- *Diminishing returns.* Up to a point, comprehensiveness improves the plan. Beyond that point, the gain is not enough to be worth the cost.
- *Technology.* Examine only those areas that can be measured by established technical and mathematical tools readily available to you.
- *Ideology.* If your ideology says a human is an economic animal, it automatically eliminates all noneconomic human elements.

The key *pitfall* of reduction is as obvious as its advantages: what you leave out diminishes your accuracy. If the omissions are marginal, the degree of error is not great enough to affect the planning.

However, serious omissions can subvert a plan. When the Pruitt-Igoe housing project in St. Louis was built, it was hailed as a model low-income housing plan. A generation later, "Pruitt-Igoe" was synonymous with the worst inner-city problems and government bungling. The reason: it never occurred to the planners to consider sociocultural factors. While the housing itself was fully standard, the side effects were disastrous. It razed, and did not replace, such traditional community-building institutions as front stoops, play areas (the street) that could be supervised from parents' windows, the corner candy store, and the bodega or deli. Unlike upper-class, high-rise urbanites, the local neighborhood was a primary social support system for these residents. Sociologists called the project's effect "social disorganization."

"How does one translate complexity into simplicity without falling into the trap of mistaking the model for the reality itself?" (Hudson, 1979, p. 392). There is no infallible way to avoid simplification mistakes, but the surest way to guarantee them is an arrogant belief in the infallibility of one's technology. If this is unwitting, it is even more dangerous, for errors are less likely to be caught along the way.

Break It Down: Deconstruction

Says Merkhofer (1987, p. 57), "Decision-aiding approaches are all based on the concept of divide and conquer." Major planning projects are too complex to handle all in one piece. We must somehow cut them into chewable bites.

A classical approach has been *deconstructionism*, a belief that the properties and functions of any complex whole can be fully explained in terms of the units of which it is made up. Its origin is Descartes' Second Maxim for science and mathematics (1637), "to break down every problem into as many separate, simple elements as might be possible." He included living organisms, and his successors applied it to social systems as well.

The method is clear-cut. Break it down into component parts. Continue to break down those components into subparts and sub-subparts as far as feasible. Analyze and intervene with each part separately. The whole is neither more nor less than the sum of its parts.

This may work in dealing with an old car with low power, poor mileage, and stalling and starting problems: clean, retime, or replace the plugs and points as necessary; adjust the carburetor; replace dirty air, oil, and gasoline filters; check the fuel pump—repair or replace if faulty; check compression for possible cylinder leakage–replace if necessary; etc. This being an honest-to-gosh mechanical system, deconstructionism may be effective. Each part is indeed separable, and the effects of separate actions are additive.

The limitations of deconstruction appear when facing the living, dynamic, interactive dimensions of an organism or social system.

The fragmentation may lead to a host of disjointed actions that work at cross-purposes with each other and with the overall system's best interest.

Deconstructed, the Bible's panorama of unfolding revelation becomes a collection of "proof texts" taken out of context.

A deconstructionist approach to family problems might diagnose and treat each member separately, expecting each result to enhance the family. According to general systems theory, it will change the dynamics of the family. These changes may enhance the family, but they can as readily destabilize it, as is often the case for families of recovering alcoholics. This is the rationale for doing *family* therapy.

Given its limitations, when is deconstruction useful? In mechanical-technical areas and in relatively simple, highly structured settings, it may be close enough to reality to meet your planning purposes efficiently.

It may be useful in achieving limited objectives. In my college, you can plan a bachelor's degree this way. Requirements are broken into six categories: basic skills, math and science, humanities, social sciences, electives, and a major. With a few exceptions, all you have to do is take a specified number of courses from each subcategory's laundry list. Any listed course will do. Neatly deconstructed, forty discrete pieces (courses) add up to the degree. (Whether it also achieves the broader goal of a good education is another question.)

Break It Down: Decomposition

Decomposition offers many of the same advantages without the liabilities. According to Merkhofer (1987, p. 58):

> The model decomposes a complicated process into more manageable components *whose relationships are made explicit* (italics supplied). For example, a model relating alternatives to outcomes often consists of sub-models for physical, environmental, or market processes; each of these, in turn, is composed of variables representing important factors and their relationships. Thus the overall decision model is a simplified representation of the important characteristics of the system that will be affected by the decision.

First you develop a holistic overview, global, and strategic. Then you identify the key elements essential to (1) determining goals, and (2) achieving the plan.

These key elements are sorted and subdivided into *interrelated* specific segments. Continue to subdivide segments through as many stages as appropriate to increase manageability. Set clear objectives for each in the context of the total plan. Delegate responsibility for each to subplanners or units, who ideally have special expertise in that segment. Give them flexibility on means, bounded vertically by the delegated objectives and resources, and horizontally by compatibility with parallel segments.

Maintain holistic coordination through central accountability, monitoring, supervision, and interunit consultations. A common approach is Likert's hierarchy of linked groups. The working unit personnel meet periodically in a group led by the unit head. Each unit head meets in a group led by the larger segment leader, who in turn meets with other major segment leaders in a group led by the planning director.

At the end (better yet, continuously along the way) do *synthesis* ("combining parts, elements, or components into a complex whole that has characteristics that differ from those of the components"). This requires that the overall planners give priority to holistic perspectives even as the units are pursuing their separate tasks. The end of decomposition is recomposition.

POSITIVISM

A discussion of rationality in planning is not complete without a reference to positivism, an Age-of-Enlightenment philosophy, originated by August Comte, which believes that the only true knowledge is based solely on positive, observable, measurable, scientific facts, relating to each other according to natural law. Everything else, including thought and feeling, must be explained only in terms of these mathematical and physical laws. It has lost some of its overt appeal as a philosophy, but is "alive and well and living in Planville."

Because right and wrong cannot be measured mathematically, positivism claims to be value neutral. It "relies on a value-free social science capable of objectively probing the etiology of social problems and presenting programs for action based upon fact rather than upon institutional or other values (Rein, 1969)."

The problem with positivism in planning is that there is no pure positivism. While the "facts" themselves may be "neutral," the a priori criteria, which select what information to collect and slant its interpretation and applications, are not. Further, since planning requires choices among competing interests, it is impossible to act on a value-neutral basis. There was nothing neutral about Columbia University's decision to evict the residents of my in-laws' stable, low-income neighborhood in order to do urban renewal (for upscale housing to be used by Columbia faculty and staff). It may have been right. It may have been wrong. It may have been debatable. What it was *not* was a value-neutral inference from their extensive data analysis.

Does this mean we should reject all positivism in planning? Yes and no. It cannot provide normative decisions. But as long as there is a navigator on board to chart the course, a crew of positivist technicians can do an excellent job. In their place, positivist methods of measuring are invaluable to the important material side of planning.

REFERENCES

Descartes, R. (1637). *Discours de la methode.*

Hudson, B. (1979). Comparisons of current planning theories. *Journal of the American Institute of Planners*, 45, pp. 387-398.

Huxley, T. (1877), "On Elemental Instruction in Physiology." In *Bartlett's Familiar Quotations*, 13th ed. Boston: Little, Brown.

Merkhofer, M. (1987). *Decision science and social risk management.* Boston: D. Reidel.

Mills, H. (1959). *Mathematics and the managerial imagination.* Princeton: Mathematica.

National Conference of Catholic Bishops (1986). *Economic justice for all.* Washington.

Rein, M. (1969). "Social planning: The search for legitimacy." *Journal of the American Institute of Planners*, 35, pp. 233-244.

Simon, H. (1957). *Models of man.* New York: Wiley.

Steiner, G. (1979). *Strategic planning.* New York: Free Press.

Weber, M. (1958). *The Protestant ethic and the spirit of capitalism.* New York: Charles Scribner's Sons.

II. DIFFERENT APPROACHES
TO PLANNING

Sometimes it seems there are as many approaches to planning as there are planners. Since every plan is unique, and planners are both diverse and creative, this is not so far from the truth.

The differences among approaches can be clustered into four sets of planning model choices: comprehensiveness, cognitive style, decision makers, and flexibility. Each is affected by one's world-view and systems model.

One aspect of *comprehensiveness* is scope. How wide are the boundaries of this plan? Over how long a time period? To what extent are externals considered, either as input variables or as spill-over effects? Another is *exhaustiveness*. How many distinct parts are developed and coordinated? How many alternative courses of action are examined? How many variables are taken into account in choosing among them? How much data needs to be collected, and how thoroughly analyzed? How much specialized technical information is required? A third is *level of aspiration*. An aim to select and achieve the best possible result calls for a much more comprehensive approach than one which seeks only to suffice.

The two major *cognitive* ("ways of knowing") approaches are (1) systematic *empirical* analysis, which breaks down complex wholes into measurable tangibles, and (2) a broader perspective, which includes *intuition*, insight, and considered judgment.

One choice of *decision makers* is an elite ("the best part of a group, as a society or a profession"). Like Plato's ideal of the philosopher king, it relies on central decisions by those who know what is best for others. In planning, this is assumed to be expert professional planners. The other is *participation*: "Please Mother,

I'd rather do it myself." It stresses that those affected by the plan should have a say.

At one end of the *flexibility* continuum is the *blueprint* approach: make detailed plans and carry them out. It is like motorboating: gas up, open the throttle, and steer the charted course. The other end is more like sailing: chart a general course, but as you make your way, you must shift with the winds. At times this may require tacking, working your way toward the destination in a zig-zag pattern rather than a straight line. *Contingency* planning is prepared to make adjustments to different possible conditions along the way.

In this section, common planning approaches are sorted out in relation to these four sets of key choices, using a dialectic framework. The starting point thesis on each is the classical Comprehensive Rational Analytical Method (CRAM). Other approaches are presented as *antitheses* or, in some cases, as *syntheses* on one of the choices. In this simplified framework, each approach is addressed in the category which "by and large" it best fits.

Chapter 6 summarizes the origins and characteristics of the comprehensive rational planning method and the most popular anticompressive antitheses–incrementalism and satisficing–together with a mixed scanning synthesis.

Chapter 7 looks at cognitive and flexibility antitheses, which ironically criticize CRAM for being too limited. A strategic approach broadens the perspective in both goal-setting and implementation. Contingency antitheses reject the assumption of a stable future and address uncertainty through a variety of anticipatory and responsive methods.

The participatory antitheses of Chapter 8 challenge the view that elite authorities know best and act disinterestedly. They include approaches to empower nonelites and involve them in decisions which affect them.

Specific planning efforts rarely fit neatly into a single approach. This may be a good thing because each has its assets and its deficiencies. A wise plan tends to be eclectic ("made up of what is selected from diverse sources").

Chapter 6

Comprehensive or Piecemeal?

If you expect to see the final result of your work, you haven't asked the right question.

–I. F. Stone

COMPREHENSIVE RATIONAL ANALYTICAL METHOD (CRAM)

The roots of classic "CRAM" planning lie in the Age of Enlightenment's rationalism and scientific method. It has several twentieth-century roots:

- Housing and town planning, led by architects and engineers, expanded into "city beautiful" master planning, and later widened to include some social planning.
- "Scientific management" in business was developed by efficiency engineers, and widened over time into the economic production model and cost-benefit analysis.
- Keynesian theories of supply-and-demand evolved into macro-economic planning.
- Welfare Economics blended macro economics and cost-benefit analysis into a collectivist social planning model.

Characteristics

Classic planning has a unitary-collective worldview. The whole transcends the special interests of any part. Operating from a closed mechanistic systems model, it approaches a stable and predictable world by breaking it down into component parts within a rationally structured master design.

> The comprehensive planner must assume that his community's various collective goals can somehow be measured at least roughly as to importance and welded into a single hierarchy of community objectives. In addition he must argue that technicians like himself can prescribe courses of action to achieve those objectives without great distortion or harmful side effects of a magnitude sufficient to outweigh the gains achieved through planning. (Altschuler, 1965)

CRAM is:

- *Synoptic:* "taking a general view of the whole or of the principal parts of a subject."
- *Comprehensive:* "inclusive, of large scope; having a wide mental grasp." It sets broad goals from which specific objectives and actions are deduced.
- *Coordinating:* "to place or arrange in due order or proper relative position."
- *Consistent:* "agreement among themselves of the parts of a complex thing," both vertically with the broad goal and horizontally with each other.

CRAM assumes the ability to do comprehensive data analysis:

- *Availability* of an extensive, adequate data base.
- *Resources* to collect and process it exhaustively.
- *Technical capacity* to analyze it scientifically.
- *Time* to complete such an analysis before making decisions.

CRAM believes that technician-planners have a detached objectivity. They are "value neutral" and disinterested, just following where the "facts" lead them. This, in combination with their technical skills, uniquely qualifies them to know better than anyone else what is best for the organization, community, or target group.

CRAM also assumes the power and resources to carry it out,

either directly or through access to others who will read, listen, understand, and respond rationally to the planners.

A Simple CRAM Model

1. Receive "given" normative guidelines (what is desirable) before the planning begins. They may be explicitly given by a sponsor or implicitly taken for granted as "self-evident" or "emerging from the data."
2. Identify and define the plan's boundaries: geographic, demographic, subject areas. Gather information for a preliminary appraisal of the situation, and based on this, set the overall goal.
3. Do a detailed analysis of the problem-condition. Break it down into component pieces.
4. For each piece, elaborate all possible specific objectives. Compare them on how much each contributes to the master goal. Keep the best ones for further analysis.
5. For each objective selected, elaborate all possible alternative means to achieve it. Evaluate each alternative on three criteria: effectiveness, feasibility, and efficiency.
6. Based on this analysis, choose the best shot. This may be one objective, a cluster of interdependent objectives, or, if you have the resources, several parallel ones.
7. Develop a detailed implementation design which schedules and coordinates the various activities required. This includes delegating responsibility, providing for needed resources, and establishing mechanisms to monitor, coordinate, and evaluate.

Linear Programming

A high-tech version of CRAM involves a mathematical model called linear programming. "The technique is intended to reveal the course of intervention leading to the best possible result, to specify how the individual parts should behave in order to maintain consistency and make the total system optimal" (Augustinovics, 1975). A simplified summary:

1. Identify the data needed and the formulae for processing them.
2. Collect quantitative data. (Qualitative data must be converted to quantitative indicators or ignored.)

3. Using this data, calculate for each possible course of action the cost of doing it, the value of its outcome if successful, and its probability of succeeding.
4. Mathematically identify the single optimum "solution" to that particular "problem."

Who Uses CRAM?

This is a preferred model for physical planning, central-command economies, and military war games. For many years it was the model of choice for rational corporate planning too, but has been modified by some of the antitheses to be discussed later. It also works well for finite subplanning, such as for a highway segment within the interstate system or for a project management design to implement an already-selected objective.

It is most effective where the following conditions exist:

- A stable, predictable environment. It is not for turbulence or rapid change.
- A structured situation where variables and relationships are well-known, specifiable, and controllable.
- High consensus among actors on desirable outcomes, facts, and feasibility. It is not for a plural-competitive worldview.
- The planning subject is tangible, with few human-element "curves."

Criticisms

The antithesis is two similar approaches, *incrementalism* and *satisficing*. CRAM overcomplicates the planning process with its massive structure and its proliferation of alternatives, many of which could have been ignored or dismissed out of hand. It carries analysis beyond what will actually be used in practice.

It faces a "Catch 22." On the one hand, it doesn't have full information, so it needs more data. On the other hand, it already has more variables and more data than it can digest.

Further, however comprehensive, all data is weakened by the fact that it is about the *past*, whereas the plan will unfold in an unknowable *future*. The uncertainty of predictions based on the past increases with the longevity of a plan.

Given human fallibility, planners are going to make mistakes. A big, broad plan makes big, broad mistakes, which are exacerbated when the planner does not recognize his or her limitations. It is safer to take it a step at a time. When you make an incremental mistake, it is a small one that can be rectified before it goes any further.

Then there is the matter of cost. Exhaustive analysis is expensive. The law of diminishing returns is operating. The first basic information you gather is cheap and makes a big improvement in your planning. An increase in data collection and analysis costs more and gains less than the first level, but it may still be worth it. Beyond some point, it costs more to do the analysis than the value of its contribution, siphoning off money from more productive uses. It also takes too long.

There is a tide in the affairs of men
Which, taken at the flood, leads on to fortune;
Omitted, all the voyage of their life
Is bound in shallows and in miseries.

—Shakespeare
Julius Caesar

Decisions often can't wait until you have assembled all the ideally desirable data. Better to act on what you have than to miss the tide. Even when time is no problem, the longer you take to analyze data, the more obsolete it becomes.

CRAM is overoptimistic about ability to carry out a master plan. In the real world, it comes up against indifference, limited understanding, and vested interests. "The model is undesirable because it does not reflect the way decisions are actually made in government or in large scale organizations. Since incrementalism is the process that is practiced, incrementalism is the theory that should be taught" (Mayer, 1985, p. 42).

Finally, CRAM unrealistically separates ends and means, first determining where to go and then figuring out how to get there. Why waste time on goals you could not accomplish anyway?

DISJOINTED INCREMENTALISM

In "The Science of Muddling Through," Charles Lindblom (1959) unveiled his antithesis to CRAM, *Successive Limited Comparisons*, or more informally, *disjointed incrementalism*, which is:

1. *Limited.* It settles for a few already familiar alternatives, and explores only some of the more important possible consequences of each.
2. *Remedial.* In common with the traditional medical model, it has "a greater analytical preoccupation with ills to be remedied than positive goals to be sought. Just fix problems through a limited number of minor changes" (Gregg, 1992). I call this the DRAB principle: Don't Respond if it Ain't Broke.
3. *Disjointed.* It rejects the integrated collective system worldview in favor of a *dis*-integrated pluralism. There is no ultimate, overall goal. It addresses each problem separately without continuity or consistency.
4. *Incremental.* It starts with the status quo and makes choices only around the edges, ignoring systemic causes and interventions. It is the opposite of exhaustive. Only a small number of alternatives, with small differences between each other and between them and the starting point, are given a small review on a small number of variables with a small amount of data from experience or near at hand. Stick to the specific and concrete. Don't take off into the wild blue yonder.
5. *Modest.* It aims low, willing to settle for "good enough."
6. *Adaptive.* It is flexible, fluid, exploratory, a succession of trials, errors, and new trials.
7. *Relativist.* It substitutes *preferences*, which are competing self-interests, for transcendent values as a guide. Decisions are made on a market basis, determined by bargaining and political maneuvering, called *partisan mutual adjustment.* "The resolution of a conflict over two values is not expressed as a principle. It is best expressed by stating how much of one value is worth sacrificing to achieve an increment of another (Sillince, 1986, p. 54).

8. *Participatory* up to a point. Decisions are made by give-and-take among established "players." There is, however, no provision for assuring full or equal participation.
9. *Retrospective.* Evaluation of values takes place after the actual consequences of the trade-offs are observed. This feedback informs future trade-off negotiations. Success is not evaluated against a goal but rather by the difference between "before" and "after."

SATISFICING

Criticism of Maximizing

An anticomprehensive approach related to disjointed incrementalism was developed at about the same time by Herbert Simon (1957a), in reaction to a business sector CRAM approach called maximizing, which used quantitative analysis to find the best possible payoff, taking into account the value of the intended result, the probability of achieving it, and the cost of doing so.

Simon criticized its aura of absolute, definitive, scientific authority and its substitution of data analysis for common sense. In its quest for precise data, it passed over important qualitative elements and judgments. For all its precise processes, its data was incomplete and often unreliable. It was out of touch with the realities of managerial decision making:

> The logic of theory arranges the stages of decision as an orderly, rational process, moving from the setting of objectives to the determination of the final course of action to be taken. It has symmetry, logic and a beginning and an end.

> The logic of *practice* is made up by the time and interest of the executive, his pressures, and the day-to-day judgments on numerous decisions which he goes through in a single day. He makes a fragmentary judgment on a single part of a larger problem, then awaits further developments. He seldom has time to stick with one major problem to carry it through two or more stages of action. . . . He is more like a juggler than a weight lifter. (Odiorne, 1965)

Characteristics

Simon's answer was, "the replacement of the goal of maximizing with the goal of *satisficing*, or finding a course of action that is 'good enough' . . . this substitution is an essential step in the application of the principle of bounded rationality" (1957b, p. 205). This approach includes nonscientific intuitive and heuristic methods, and leans toward incremental caution.

PROS AND CONS

Advantages

As noted, incrementalism is a hedge against major mistakes and abuse of power by central planners. While it may not maximize from the point of view of a unitary-collective system, its balancing of competing values, interests, and preferences may work better in plural-collaborative circumstances.

Incremental plans may succeed more often. Changes which, in a single step, would bring down the wrath of vested interests, may be accepted an inch at a time.

Its nonjudgmental stance is attractive to those who value client self-determination. It "recognizes that planners do not have to determine what is 'right'" (Valentine, 1991).

When is incremental satisficing most desirable?

- When a quick fix is needed.
- When there is neither time nor money for extensive review of all possibilities.
- When interim adjustments are needed to buy time for long-range planning.
- When a major fundamental decision is not needed—or not wanted. The existing situation is relatively satisfactory and does not need major changes.

Common settings for incrementalism include politics, bureaucracy, business and program administration, collaboration, conflict negotiation, social casework, decentralized operations, and personal planning.

Criticisms

This approach leans toward the lowest common denominator of acceptability. This is rarely the best choice and often a poor one. "Its main impact is an ideological reinforcement of the pro-inert and anti-innovation forces" (Dror, 1964).

It is inherently *conservative* in its uncritical de facto endorsement of whatever the current status quo may be, good or bad. It does not lift a finger to transcend or transform it. Its bounded rationality might more accurately be called a "bounded *pessimism*" which is too hasty to discount nonconventional courses which a "bounded optimism" might discover.

> Incrementalism tends to neglect basic societal innovations, as it focuses on the short run and seeks no more than limited variations from past policies. While an accumulation of small steps could lead to a significant change, there is nothing in this approach to guide the accumulation. (Etzioni, 1967)

It undervalues side effects that can make a difference in the costs and/or benefits of a plan. It may narrowly choose a less desirable plan by ignoring spillovers, especially ones affecting bystanders who weren't "at the planning table."

Some planning tasks, such as public transit in New York City, nuclear power plants, saving the Everglades, or a universal health care system do not lend themselves to incremental planning. On a personal level, the surest way to end up with an ABD (All But Dissertation) is to pursue a PhD inch by inch.

In some cases, seemingly marginal incremental decisions can have major and irreversible consequences. For instance, if a number of fragmented improvements in roadways encourage some commuters to switch from public transit or to move farther out, the result may be even more traffic congestion.

Planners with a strong social commitment criticize this antithesis as amoral in its substitution of preferences and competition for a priori values. There is no right or wrong. "What is acceptable is good" (Scurfield, 1992).

SYNTHESES

Upgraded Satisficing

An unflattering acronym for satisficing is SOSO (Slough Off to Sub Optimization). Some business planners wanted to keep the common sense approach of satisfice, yet do more than just get by. They found a middle ground by upgrading "satisfice" from adequacy to the best practical choice under the circumstances, while the optimizers softened the rigidity of their position.

> The object of an optimizing analysis is [not] to find the best of *all* possible courses of action; such a task is hopeless. . . . Only after a set of "reasonable contenders" has thus been defined does it become possible to apply formal procedures for choices among them. . . . "Satisficing" is as good a word as any to denote both the preliminary choice of contenders and the intuitive elimination of some of them. (Raiffa and Schlaifer, 1961)

Rejointed Incrementalism

Twenty years after presenting disjointed incrementalism, Lindblom (1979) conceded the advantages of organizing increments into a strategic framework:

> The corrective is . . . the supplementation of incremental analysis by broad-ranging, often highly speculative and sometimes utopian thinking. . . . A fast moving sequence of small changes can more speedily accomplish a drastic alteration of the status quo than can an only infrequent major policy change.

The key word is *sequence*, "a continuous or related series of things following in a certain order."

Mixed Scanning

Amatai Etzioni's *mixed scanning* (1967) developed the classic synthesis of comprehensive and incremental. It seeks to correct such CRAM "faults" as:

- Positivist reductionism to the exclusion of the human element.
- The diminishing returns of exhaustiveness.
- The value vacuum.
- Ignoring political and power realities.
- Unrealistic expectations about being able to collect all data necessary for a comprehensive rational choice within the reality of an unlimited open system of variables.

At the same time, it avoids incrementalist pitfalls:

- Lack of overall perspective, direction, or purpose.
- Expedient "fixes" which ignore fundamental problems.
- Disjointed fragmentation.
- Missing better alternatives due to superficial analysis.

Mixed scanning has two levels of scope. The "fundamental" or "broad" is "all-encompassing." This corresponds to the global and strategic levels in our BASIC model. The "incremental" or "bit" deals with BASIC's tactical and operational levels.

It selectively blends from both CRAM and incremental methods. Any number of alternative courses of action may be identified, but instead of an obsessively detailed overall analysis, it permits a "truncated" scan which boils them down to a few live options, within the context of which a detailed analytical review may be used to evaluate and choose among specific objectives and means, particularly in regard to feasibility, tactics, and implementation design.

CRAM is accused of not being able to see the forest for the trees. Scanning permits an overall perspective that is neither restricted by positivist "scientific" tunnel vision nor obscured by obsessive detail.

Incrementalism is accused of being inherently conservative, never straying far from the status quo, and directionless (fragmented). This is offset by making incremental decisions within the context of the broad, longer-range perspectives of the fundamental scan. Further, mixed scanning permits comprehensive detailing of appropriate, specific incremental pieces of the action.

The actual mix of scanning and detailed analysis depends on what you need to make a decision. A quick and dirty scan may be all that is necessary where the choice is easy and clear-cut. Detailed analysis may be needed where there is ambiguity or uncertainty, as well as in dealing with the nitty-gritty of implementation. How much you already know is a factor. Old pros in familiar territory can do more scanning. Another factor is how much you are able to do. A mixed scanning perspective lets you spend your limited time and resources where they will do the most good.

Mixed scanning "corrects" the rejection of explicit values by both CRAM and incrementalism by encouraging both decision makers and other interested parties to do an informal scaling or ranking of their value priorities. (See the previous chapter on VIBES.)

REFERENCES

Altschuler, A. (1965). "The goals of comprehensive planning." *Journal of the American Institute of Planners*, 31.

Augustinovics, M. (1975). "Integration of mathematics and traditional methods of planning." In Bornstein, M., E*conomic planning: East and West*. Cambridge, MA: Ballinger, pp. 127-148.

Dror, Y. (1964). "Muddling through–'Science' or inertia?" *Public Administration Review*, 24.

Etzioni, A.(1967). "Mixed scanning: A third approach to decision making." *Public Administration Review*, 27, pp. 385-392.

Gregg, S. (1992). Unpublished paper. University of Nebraska-Omaha.

Lindblom, C. (1959). "The science of muddling through." *Public Administration Review*, 19, pp. 79-88.

Lindblom, C. (1979). "Still muddling, not yet through." *Public Admininstration Review*, 39, pp. 517-526.

Mayer, R. (1985). *Policy and program planning: A developmental perspective*. Englewood, NJ: Prentice-Hall.

Odiorne, G. (1965). *Management by objectives*. New York: Pitman.

Raiffa, H. and Schlaifer R. (1961). *Applied statistical decision theory*. Cambridge, MA: Harvard.

Scurfield, G. (1992). Unpublished paper. University of Nebraska-Omaha.

Sillince, J. (1986). *A theory of planning*. Brookfield, VT: Gower.

Simon, H. (1957a). *Administrative behavior*. New York: Macmillan.

Simon, H. (1957b). *Models of man*. New York: Wiley.

Valentine, K. (1991). Unpublished paper. University of Nebraska-Omaha.

Chapter 7

It's Not That Simple

When thou hast done, thou hast not done, for I have more.

–John Donne
"A Hymn to God the Father, 1625"

WICKED PROBLEMS

CRAM's world can be measured objectively within a consistent, finite structure. This works well in engineering, where most things can be converted to mathematical equations. It does not do so well with open social systems, which are populated by "wicked" problems. A problem is wicked when it has some or all of the following characteristics (Rittell and Webber, 1973):

- *No definitive formulation of the problem or potential solutions is possible.* It is impossible to encompass all the ever-changing elements of a live social situation with a simple mechanical cause-and-effect formula. Solutions are not neatly true or false. The judgments of diverse parties "are likely to differ widely to accord with their group or personal interests, their special value-sets, and their ideological predilections."
- *No problem is isolated.* "No man is an island, entire of itself; every man is a piece of the continent, a part of a main" (John Donne, Devotions; 1624). This insight is reflected in professional social work education's required first course: Human Behavior in the Social Environment.
- *No two cases are the same.* While we can learn much from standardized data, there is always something essentially unique in each situation that precludes a one-size-fits-all boilerplate.

For instance, although many of my colleagues treat a student plan of study that way, I have never encountered two students just alike. My job is, within the bounds of the program, to help each one tailor a plan of study to his or her particular interests and goals.

- *There is no clear finish line.* In the living, changing world of human society, you never reach the end. A plan does not end because the problem is solved once and for all, but rather when it reaches a point where the planner says, "that's good enough," or "this is the best I can do under the circumstances." There can be no ultimate test of the results: "We have no way of tracing all the waves through all the affected lives ahead of time."

Positivist Reduction

As a social planning method, say its critics, CRAM is narrowed by positivist reductionism. It "scientizes" planning through "neat, logical, and antiseptic definitions of the messy disorderly affairs of people . . . [as] computable notions" (Ewing, 1969, p. 39).

This devalues or even excludes qualitative dimensions of human life. "One reason the public have been attacking the social professions, we believe, is that the cognitive and occupational styles of the professions—mimicking the cognitive style of science and the occasional style of engineering—have just not worked on a wide array of social problems" (Rittell and Webber, 1973).

Pseudoneutrality

CRAM's claimed objectivity is unattainable. There is no critical analysis of one's own a priori assumptions and selective perceptions. The problem is exacerbated if the planners naively believe that they are objective. For instance, in dismissing a priori values, they don't seem to realize that the philosophy that colors their perceptions is itself an a priori belief, neither proven nor disproven by empirical science.

"Value neutral" planning is an oxymoron, for by definition, all planning is goal oriented. "Appropriate planning action cannot be prescribed from a position of value neutrality, for prescriptions are based on desired objects . . . . Values are inescapable elements in any rational decision-making process" (Davidoff, 1965). The result is a pseudoneutrality in which the planners project their own (or their sponsors') VIBES, follow current ideological fads, or fall into the reasoning pitfalls discussed in Chapter 5.

A Closed Mind in a Closed System

An agreement reached by the Congregational and Presbyterian churches in the early 1800s divided the country equally–at the Hudson River. The former's image of America has been described as New England, New York City, and a blue haze beyond the Hudson. Everything outside CRAM's mechanistic boundaries is a blue haze.

CORRECTIVE: STRATEGIC PLANNING

Strategic comes from the Greek word for a general. In its original form, strategic planning, alias "total overall planning," "long-range planning," "integrative planning," and British "corporate planning," has served as a "corrective" to both CRAM reductionism and incrementalist fragmentation. It adds a broader, non-bounded level to their sublunary ("earthbound") preoccupation. It determines "how the selection of decisions is made, on what principles, and for what purposes a specific choice is made, with what aim, why, how much, and where planning is taking place" (Bicanic, 1967, p. 76).

A key contribution of strategic planning is to widen the vista. "Formal strategic planning is an effort to duplicate what goes on in the mind of a brilliant intuitive planner" (Steiner, 1979, p. 10). It uses available empirical data and analysis–plus nonscience experience, insight, and educated guesses. It makes conscious VIBES choices which interact with pragmatic realities. Recognizing the fallibility of each, it affirms multiple sources. It prefers blended Scotch to a single malt.

> Emphasis . . . has shifted away from algorithmic approaches (i.e., quantitative programming and modeling techniques) and

toward integrative problem solving approaches . . . [which] are not as utopian as rationalism but not as conservative or pessimistic about the role of analysis as the classical incrementalists. . . . The complexity of emerging problems necessarily places the planner at the crossroads between analysis and politics. (Hart, 1986, p. 117)

A good strategic planner will digest this varied intelligence into a user-friendly form. "A manager prefers simple analysis that he can grasp, even though it may have a qualitative structure, broad assumptions, and only a little relevant data, to a complex model whose assumptions may be partially hidden or couched in jargon and whose parameters may be the result of obscure statistical manipulation" (Little, 1979, p. B-466).

A by-product of strategic planning's eclectic approach to gathering intelligence is a greater emphasis on involvement of informants and interested parties. Its openness increases flexibility at the tactical level and the ability to adjust to unfolding development.

SECOND-GENERATION STRATEGIC PLANNING

Originally, "strategic" was a partial-planning supplement in response to the narrowness of other planning approaches. As it became an "in" method, especially in the business sector, it spun off *strategic administration*, a multilevel process which moved the whole way from mission statement to front line actions. The outline below draws on Kulik's summary (1992):

1. *Master strategy level:* the big picture.
   A. Review the organization's purpose, mandates, and VIBES; and scan of the environment, including trends and external potential actors. Weigh current versus future responsibilities, interests, and opportunities. Evaluate its existing mission and goals in light of these analyses. Write (or revise) a *mission* statement of the organization's values, purpose, and general direction.
   B. Within the mission, define the *boundaries* of this plan. Ask the right question. Choose the right problem to solve. Iden-

tify the areas (subject, geographic, etc.). Set the fundamental broad goals.

    C. Gather strategic *intelligence* about the practicalities:
- The organization's internal characteristics, weaknesses and strengths.
- What is within your control. What is not (the environment).
- Tangible empirical facts about the existing situation, including needs- and feasibility-assessment.
- Qualitative information about the values, interests, and preferences of the actors who may affect the plan and those who may be affected by it, directly or indirectly.

    D. Develop the *master strategy,* an overall framework with guidelines and boundaries to be honored by all subsequent-level decision makers and actors. This includes the finalized fundamental goal(s) and broad courses of action or direction to get there.

2. *Program strategy level,* also called functional planning.

    A. Subdivide the plan into particular applications. This is often done through two or more successive levels, middle-range program goals and immediate unit objectives. At each level develop goals-objectives and courses of action, guided and bounded by the decision of the next "higher" (broader) level of program decision.

    B. Delegate decentralized responsibility and accountability for each application.

3. *Operational level.* Spell out actions to be taken in a designed pattern of coordinated steps. Assign responsibility for each task. Assure that resources are available. Build in feedback to monitor performance and make timely adjustments.

4. *Periodic master strategy review.* Reexamine the fundamental mission and goals, update the middle-range goals, and specify the next set of short-term objectives.

Assets and Liabilities

Second-generation strategic planning is popular because it is a synthesis of several approaches. It keeps a CRAM structure while avoiding many of its limitations. At each level, it deals with qualitative as well as quantitative elements, values, insight from experience, and is open to partisan mutual adjustment. Like mixed scanning, it is comprehensive in scope but not uptight about exhaustive analysis. It can adapt to the available level of information.

Where is it useful? It was designed for planning by large, complex organizations and is applicable to macro-planning in all sectors. At the same time, the approach can be adapted to more modest areas such as getting fit, family planning, seeking election to the school board . . . or developing a planning course.

Strategic planners are not always appreciated. In Japan, where deferred gratification is common, stockholders reward a wise corporate executive who plans strategically for long-term growth and payoff. On the other hand, American stockholders, focused on maximizing short-term returns, have been known to fire such an executive. Similarly, politicians who want to stay in office must give priority to what will please the voters before the next election. If they make strategic social investments now which will pay off in the future, they may well be gone before the benefits are felt (and some undeserving successor on whose watch the payoffs emerge reaps the credit for their foresight).

The senator in the *Shoe* comic strip understands this way of thinking. He promises voters immediate new benefits and tax cuts. "How will you pay for them?" "In the outyear budget." "What's that?" "The years after I am out of office."

LIVING WITH CHANGE

No one ever steps in the same stream twice.

—Heraclitus

Oh, we don't know what's comin' tomorrow.
Maybe it's trouble and sorrow,
But we'll travel along . . .

—Harry Woods, 1927
"Side by side"

Traditional planning develops a *blueprint* ("plan"). It assumes you know all you need to know. Once the plan is designed, get the job done.

Unrealistic, say the critics. Despite our best efforts–and we *should* try–the real-world environment remains complex, vaguely defined, incompletely known, and inconsistent. And it does not stand still. As we go along, we discover new things: updated needs assessment, information about the VIBES of stakeholders, additional empirical data, preliminary results. Meanwhile changes in the "environment" occur, affecting (for good and ill) the feasibility of specific objectives, means, and designs.

LEARNING-ADAPTIVE PROCESS (LAP)

A plan is out of date by the time it is in use.

Ewing, 1969

LAP's systems model is based on a living organism: fluid, adaptive, constantly growing and changing. It is the antithesis of a blueprint. "Unfolding intelligence" comes through "social practice . . . the interplay of knowing and doing" (Friedman, 1979). This enables the planner to revise the "image" of the system, on the basis of which midstream adjustments are continuously made. Critics counter that LAP's goals tend to be fuzzy and its shifting sands subvert effective goal-directed action.

It optimistically works toward consensus among diverse actors through persuasion, education, voluntary accommodation, and give-and-take tradeoffs, as opposed to CRAM's "thinking head, servile limbs." In the process, it mixes together facts, assumptions, theories, feelings, and value judgments. Its proponerets call it a blending. Others say it is a jumble.

While LAP may be naive as a primary model for a complex macro-planning project, it may be very effective at the micro level, such as a family or a parish society. Perhaps its greatest value, however, lies as a selectively applied technique within other planning approaches.

CONTINGENCY PLANNING

A *contingency* is "something whose occurrence depends on chance and uncertain events." Health insurance is a contingency measure. So is saving for a rainy day.

"Contingency planning should eliminate fumbling, uncertainty, and time delays in making the needed response to an emergency. Contingency planning also should make successful responses more rational" (Steiner, 1979, p. 230).

It prepares for uncontrollable events along the way. Since the future never can be predicted with certainty, all information and assumptions about expected circumstances are at best probabilities. These may be estimated by comprehensive rational analysis, intuition, and/or a blend of both, called "decision theory." (See Chapter 19.)

Key assumptions about elements not under our control, such as the behavior of various actors, resources available, the state of the economy, etc., are made explicit. Indicators are developed to tell if they change. When they do, the assumptions are revised and the plan altered accordingly.

This is not so much a "model" as an "approach" that can be blended into most planning models.

Adaptiveness

Key for any adaptive method is a master strategy, a clear sense of where you are, where you want to go, and why. One ingredient is to be clear on the broad mission and direction. Another is to have thought out your value-interest-preference hierarchy and how it affects priorities within the plan: what is essential, what is secondary, and what is expendable.

Add a flexible, creative *mindset*, and stir. Contributing to this are socialization and experience, which make it second nature to anticipate possible futures and to be innovative in response to the unexpected. I call it imagineering. It flourishes where people are praised and rewarded for good ideas, not only when they pay off but also for "good tries." A series of Hewlett-Packard commercials presented the company in this mode: a variety of employees each getting a bright idea at the beach, walking the dog, etc., and rushing to the nearest phone to call the boss (whom they obviously expect to be pleased by such an intrusion). The scene fades out with the employee saying, "*What if . . .* " According to Peters and Waterman (1982), HP really did behave that way. This does not happen in a negative bureaucracy (or family) that stresses conformity and obedience: "Don't stick your neck out. You may get it chopped off."

Built-in Tolerance

One contingency approach is to allow some leeway. In long-range planning, such as highways, airports, and water-sewage infrastructure, the tolerance may be built in by setting an excess-capacity objective at the outset.

Leeway can provide for Murphy's Law: "If anything can go wrong, it will." Planners often make three projections: high (optimistic), low (pessimistic), and middle (most likely). Conventional planning usually chooses the middle assumption.

Cautious contingency takes the low road, overbudgeting resources, time, etc., to allow the unexpected. It may also lower the risk of your looking bad, and may even get you more brownie points than if you had projected accurately and come out on target. The cost of this may be lowered efficiency. Parkinson's Law (1957) says, "Work expands so as to fill the time available for its completion." People live up or down to expectations. In one course I set a project deadline. All met it without difficulty except one who had an honest-to-gosh emergency. The next year, I set the same date but allowed a penalty-free extra week "only if it is absolutely necessary." Two-thirds needed it.

"Wouldst thou both eat thy cake and have it?" (George Herbert, *The Size;* 1663). The trick is to achieve leeway without depressing performance. One way is the gentle subterfuge of preparing two versions of the plan: a pessimistic one for public consumption while operating in fact on a private middle-to-stretch one.

A more conventional device is to develop the plan on the most probable projection, but set up a slush fund (politely known as "unallocated reserve") to dip into in a pinch. If it is not needed, it is rolled over as a reserve for the next project. For instance, my university sets aside a percentage of its overhead allowance on all grants to cover special contingencies that may arise unexpectedly in any one of them. Of course, there remains an opportunity cost: what you didn't do with those resources because you held them aside.

When the objective is important enough, *redundancy* can be

used, a full backup system in case the primary course of action hits a snag, as in the design of a nuclear power plant. On a simple level, a student applies to an Ivy League school with expectations of being accepted, but applies also to a good sure-thing backup.

A variation on this is to *duplicate*. Simultaneously pursue parallel primary courses of action. Peters and Waterman (1982) recommend competing research and development teams in large corporations. Not only does this double the chance of success, but the competition spurs each team to work harder. Eventually, only the more successful one is retained. Reforesters do this too. They plant twice as many trees as can be sustained, and cull the weaker ones when they are half-grown.

Updating Mechanisms

Contingency planning can be built into the core structure and design of the plan, such as:

- Routine monitoring of key assumptions, especially in the external environment, planning's "DEW line." (In the pre-satellite era, the United States and Canada maintained a Distant Early Warning [DEW] radar line inside the Arctic Circle to give us lead time to mobilize our response to a Russian missile attack.)
- Structured feedback links. This includes such common tools as reports, staff meetings, and management "walkarounds."
- An open-door policy encouraging new information or insight from any source, internal or external.

When there is a significant change, loop back and do a fresh strategic scan (or detailed analysis in the rare case). Revise the strategic level if necessary. Re-look at the goals, objectives, and means in light of the change. Consider revisions or alternatives that might have become desirable and feasible due to the change. This is not just problem solving. It can also be a response to a new opportunity.

The dialectic approach is useful for this analysis: the existing plan (thesis), unexpected variations from what we projected (antithesis), and an adaptive solution (synthesis).

Sunset laws are a structured contingency provision in long-range planning. When authorizing a program, the legislature adds a rider that the program automatically expires at the end of five years unless rejustified and renewed. In my professional field, accreditation is granted for a seven-year period. In the seventh year, assessors return for a new "zero base" review. You better believe we do an "awesome" self-review in the sixth year!

A more flexible structured approach is the *rolling plan*. For example, develop a five-year strategic plan, and within it, the specific objectives-means course of action for the first year. Toward the end of that first year, evaluate the specific results and review the whole picture. Based on the results and any new circumstances, revise and extend it into a new five-year plan, complete with the coming year's specific objectives and means.

Sequential Approaches

The *flow chart* is a sequential contingency blueprint. It lays out in advance each point at which alternative outcomes are possible, with a different next step for each. When the event occurs, plug in that alternative's prescribed next step.

This works well for predictable circumstances. It does not prepare for unanticipated "surprises." A rollover-style may help to resolve this problem. Instead of laying out all contingency next steps at the outset, stop, reassess, and determine the second step after you arrive at the end of step one. Taking into account the revised and updated circumstances, choose the best available course toward your master goal.

In my winter trip from Nebraska to Florida, the first step is I-29 to Kansas City. When I get there, I figure out three second-step choices: to St. Louis, Memphis, or Little Rock. Taking everything into account, I choose Memphis. On arrival, I check the current weather, the road conditions, and the forecast, then decide whether to proceed via Nashville and Atlanta, Birmingham and Montgomery, or Jackson and Mobile. And so forth.

Plan B

The most comprehensive contingency method is two (or more) *fully-developed parallel plans*. Plan A is based on the accepted key assumptions. Then Plan B is developed from the same data, based on a different contingency set of assumptions. In planning for World War III, the military does this. (Tom Clancy's novel, *Red Storm Rising*, played out one of these plans.) This is most effective when Plan A assumptions are somewhat uncertain and the probability of B assumptions is also fairly high. Plan B may be:

- A parallel, full-planning process based on the second most likely set of assumptions.
- An opportunity "wish list." Plan A is based on expected resources. The more ambitious Plan B kicks in if they exceed expectations.
- A less ambitious plan in case the A expectations don't come through.
- One of three plans premised, respectively, on the three standard projections mentioned earlier: high, average, low.
- An expedient choice among approximately equal objectives. At one time I had three tactical plans for my program's curriculum within a goal of teaching social workers ethnic diversity. Plan A was an African-American culture course, for this was our largest subgroup in our state. Plan B was Latino, and a Plan C was Native American (the smallest subgroup). An outstanding Native American professor became available. We shifted immediately from Plan A to Plan C as the coming year objective.

One can do a half-way Plan B. Instead of two full plans, develop only a schematic, broad-brush Plan B (and sometimes C and D). This way you don't waste time on the detail of something you may never use, yet it is available to be fleshed out on short notice—and it will then be fresher than a full Plan B which needs updating.

Note: In my experience, few colleagues and fewer bosses have wanted to address contingency plans. If you encounter this, plan for contingencies anyway, but keep it in a personal file. The same folks who are annoyed if you raise contingency concerns will be delighted when you (tactfully, of course) bail them out.

REFERENCES

Bicanic, R. (1967). *Problems of planning East and West.* Hague: Mouton.

Davidoff, P. (1965). "Advocacy and pluralism in planning." *Journal of the American Institute of Planners,* 31, pp. 331-338.

Ewing, D. (1969). *The human side of planning: Tool or tyrant?* New York: Macmillan.

Friedman, J. (1979). "Theory of meta-planning: Innovation, flexible response and social learning." In Burchell, R. and Sternlieb, G. (Eds.) *Planning theory in the 1980s.* New Brunswick: Center for Urban Policy Review.

Hart, S. (1986). "Planning as a strategic social process." In Dluhy, M. and Chen, K. (Eds.) *Interdisciplinary planning.* New York: Center for Urban Policy Research.

Kulick, A. (1992). Unpublished paper. University of Nebraska-Omaha.

Little, J. (1979). "Models and managers: The concept of a decision calculus." *Management Science,* 4, p. B-466.

Parkinson, C. N. (1957). *Parkinson's law.* Cambridge, MA: Riverside.

Peters, T. and Waterman, R. (1982). *In search of excellence.* New York: Warner.

Rittell, H. and Webber, M. (1973). "Dilemmas of a general theory of planning." *Policy Sciences,* 4, pp. 133-145.

Steiner, G. (1979). *Strategic planning.* New York: Free Press.

Chapter 8

Vox Populi

Vox populi, vox dei.
[The voice of the people is the voice of God.]

—Letter to Charlemagne, 800 A.D.

CRITICISM OF CRAM

The people have little intelligence.
The great have no heart.
If I have to choose, I prefer the people.

—Jean de la Bruyere, 1690
Des Grandes

All professions are conspiracies against the laity.

—George Bernard Shaw
The Doctor's Dilemma; 1906

CRAM operates on a unitary-collective worldview that believes there is an objective, knowable "general interest," which planners are best equipped to determine through data analysis. "Father knows best." Involving "the people" directly is a disorderly intrusion that muddies the water. Not so, say a diverse array of critics.

The plural-collaborative worldview defines general interest as the result of uncoerced give-and-take compromises among the preferences of "players around a table." It cannot be determined in absolute terms by some formula. Models: traditional politics and partisan mutual adjustment.

The more pessimistic plural-competitive view assumes that everyone is out for himself or herself. CRAM's so-called objectivity is in fact no more than promotion of the interests of established subgroups and their hired planners in the guise of a spurious general interest. You must protect your own interests. Model: advocacy planning.

The libertarian view favors compartmentalized self-determination. Forget general interest stuff. Let subgroups plan and act for themselves. Models: community organization and transactive planning.

POLITICAL PLANNING

The people are the masters.

—Edmund Burke, 1780

"Planning is an essentially political process because it deals with the allocation of resources. Thus ends are in question, and decisions are ultimately a matter of judgment. These decisions are taken by an exercise of power" (Cowan, 1979, p. 5).

In his city planning experience, Banfield (1955) encountered a gap between CRAM planning and political decision making. His accommodation was to *add* a political component to the CRAM model: "Where there is a conflict, real or apparent, between the ends of different actors . . . an *issue* exists. . . . *Politics* is the activity (negotiation, argument, discussion, application of force, persuasion, etc.) by which an issue is agitated or settled."

He identified several decision-making approaches:

> *Contention* . . . the parties mutually endeavor to make their ends prevail over those of the other parties, their adversaries, by the exercise of power . . . through struggle or bargaining . . .
> *Dictation* . . . one party compels the other to accept a settlement on his terms . . .
> *Cooperation* . . . the parties make a shared end (or ends), or

some procedural principle which is mutually agreed upon, the basis of the choice among the ends which are at issue . . .
Accommodation . . . one party freely chooses to make the ends of the other his own if he exacts a quid pro quo.

PARTISAN MUTUAL ADJUSTMENT

Partisan Mutual Adjustment is part of Lindblom's incrementalism model (1959,1968). It is pragmatic rather than ideological. There are multiple actors who have power to affect the plan: sponsors and authorizers, funders, vested interests, professionals, other staff, cooperating agencies, and consumers who have the power to accept or reject the product.

This is a *market* process. As price is negotiated between buyers and sellers, so are planning decisions reached through direct bargaining, exchange, and compromise among competing interests. It can also be done through *implicit bargaining*, in which the planner assesses each actor's preferences and priorities, and deftly tailors a proposal geared to what the traffic will bear. The planner is a broker and mediator, not a protagonist. The test of a "good" plan is acceptance, which is often defined as absence of active dissent.

GRASSROOTS EMPOWERMENT

In the people was my trust,
And in the virtues which mine eyes had seen.

—Wordsworth
"The Prelude"

Two recognized grassroots planning approaches are:

- Group *Advocacy* Planning (GAP), which tries to fill the gap in the policy arena for persons who have been left out.
- *Transactive* Adaptive Planning (TAP), which seeks to tap the roots of a community for self-help and mutual assistance.

The traditional political solutions of Banfield and Lindblom, say these folk, are an inadequate corrective to CRAM's association with power elites. While they do widen participation to include a diversified set of power centers in the community, they don't make any particular effort to involve under-represented interests. In retrospect, Lindblom (1979) himself acknowledged the truth of this.

Community Organization

Both GAP and TAP have their origin in traditional planners' discovery of a related field, *Community Organization* (CO), which was developed in the nineteenth century by the settlement house movement. Its aim was to empower inner-city immigrants both for self-help and for political action. It initiated cooperative projects, among them credit unions and day care, and also promoted unionization of workers and political mobilization. By 1901, it had become a master's-level Social Work specialization at the University of Chicago.

In the 1930s, Saul Alinsky (Finks, 1984; Horwitt, 1989) turned away from crimonology and social work, both of which had become too "established" and moved to community organization's roots, organizing poor people in the back of the stockyards neighborhood of Chicago to gain more control of their lives. From this beginning, he established a national CO effort through his Industrial Areas Foundation.

In the 1950s and 1960s, CO methods were adopted by many civil rights and social justice movements. About the same time, it became the core of a series of Ford Foundation Gray Cities projects such as Mobilization for Youth, which in turn were the models for the War on Poverty's Community Action Programs. Paul Davidoff (1965), a planner with a strong social justice orientation, became involved in this effort. Drawing from its CO and its legal advocacy for the poor, he came up with GAP, in which planners would work for and with "the people." While its formal applications were often naive, and its support base eroded in the Nixon-Reagan era, it remains a residual dimension in planning thought.

Meanwhile, as decolonization occurred after World War II, CO methods were applied in United Nations third-world *community development* projects. Although its wider application was subverted by authoritarian national governments and by international geopolitics, a number of local projects were highly successful. After visiting such a project, John Friedman (1973) blended CO with planning (as well as adult education theory and a bit of Zen) into a provocative transactional planning model. While rarely employed as the primary model, its methods have been used selectively in many planning efforts.

There are two streams of CO. The *traditional* approach is nondirective. It draws out feelings and wants, then helps the members to express them, work through them, and act on them. In the introduction to his classic, *Organizing*, Si Kahn (1991, p. 3) says:

> Early social workers who were organizing and working with groups were careful to define their role as enabling individuals to come together and develop their own leadership and decision making structure. In this enabler role, they recognized the importance of starting where the group was and becoming less central as the group developed over time.

Tactical CO uses a similar group process, except that the goal comes first, then participants who agree with it are recruited. Thereafter, the role of the organizer is to provide technical and process assistance to enable the group itself to select and carry out specific objectives and actions within the shared goal.

These two types can be combined. Si Kahn spends the first half of his book on traditional CO and then devotes the second half to tactical CO. In his own practice, he made the two compatible by doing traditional CO, but only with groups whose interests already coincided with his personal social justice values.

Group Advocacy Planning

An advocate is "one who pleads the cause of another."

Advocacy planning's worldview is unequivocally plural-competitive. All planning affects competing interests. No one can represent all interests. Self-interest rules; power decides. As George Bernard Shaw put it in "Maxims for Revolutionaries", "The golden rule is that there are no golden rules." Therefore, "polycentered" planning is required. Each special interests subgroup must plan independently for itself and then fight for that plan in the arena with other subgroups. One might call this "tooth and fang" planning.

All organized special interests groups do advocacy planning. The cigarette industry plans its advertising and lobbying to maximize smoking without reference to its health effects. Health advocates work to minimize the hazards of smoking without reference to Phillip Morris' profits. The established vested interests have been doing advocacy planning all along: corporations, the military, unions, builders, realtors, professional associations, chambers of commerce, political leadership.

According to GAP planners, this is proper except for two key problems. One is the con game of doing advocacy planning under the aegis of "general" welfare or the "common" interest. CRAM planning makes such claims. The other is that many subgroups, probably comprising the majority of all Americans, are excluded because they lack their own effective advocacy planning.

Subgroups, particularly those at the short end of the stick, must *counterplan* to compete with those with established advocacy planning resources. These counterplans should be more than a negative reaction to the established plan after the fact. They should be *anticipatory*. Prepare in advance so that it is ready to go as soon as the issue arises.

Better, they should be *preemptive*. Get there first, before others' thoughts have jelled, to set the framework in which others will respond. Practice "*Burch's Law*": "The first draft is 85 percent of the final decision." I "discovered" this law as the Labor Department staffer who prepared the first draft of the plan for a new program, after which I received it back to write the final version. The plan was tinkered with by four layers of approvers, who made perhaps a hundred detailed changes, but they had left the core intact. The reason is simple. Few decision makers have the time, competence, or inclination to do a major overhaul, so their review is incremental. (Note: the effect is much weaker, but not entirely absent, when the initiative conflicts with powerful vested interests.)

GAP has been ambiguous about planning with and planning for the group. Its ideology is "with": the planner provides technical assistance to the group in developing its own planning capabilities. However, CRAM-trained planners, socialized to doing technical tasks and providing directive inputs, can be awkward and insensitive in the role of nondirective enabler. So where the rubber hits the road, GAP tends to lean toward the more comfortable *lawyer* role model of planning *for.*

> The legal advocate must *plead* (italics supplied) for his own and his client's sense of legal propriety or justice. . . . The advocate planner would be responsible to his client and would seek to express his client's view. . . . He would be responsible to his client for preparing plans for all the . . . elements comprising the planning process. . . . The advocate's most important function would be to carry out the planning process for the organization and to argue persuasively in favor of its planning proposals. (Davidoff, 1965)

Since the turn away from "power to the people" after the 1960s, the "pure" GAP projects Davidoff envisioned have been rare. However, advocacy planning is still active in several ways:

- Public interest advocacy—for groups such as the Children's Defense Fund.
- Participatory methods used within broader planning models.
- Technical assistance requested by self-directed community organizations.
- Addition of a CO professional to traditional planning staffs. In my city, the Housing Authority recently hired a macro social worker to work with its tenants both for self-help and to get their inputs for future planning.

Transactive Planning

Transact means "to carry through negotiations to a settlement." The aim of transactive adaptive planning is to overcome the chasm between the planner and the planned-for.

Rooted as it is in CO, it embraces the social work principle, "start where the client is." Describing his rural Chilean model, John Friedman (1973) reported, "At the start, the newly recruited advisor spent from six months to a year learning about the multifaceted situation in which he had been placed."

TAP stresses *mutual learning* through *dialogue*:

> Transactive planning is carried on the ground swell of dia-
> logue. . . . In mutual learning, planner and client each learns
> from the other–the planner from the client's personal knowl-
> edge, the client from the planner's technical expertise. In this
> process the knowledge of both undergoes a major change.
> (Friedman, 1973)

Transactive skills are taught in adult education, social work,
educational psychology, and counseling. There are two key variations of the transactive style. One is *nondirective*, a purely enabling
method developed by therapist Carl Rogers (1951). You approach
the "client" with an open mind, acceptance, and support:

- Listen carefully.
- Repeat back what you heard or probe gently, "Do you
  mean . . . ?"
- Client clarifies, restates, rebuts, explains, or revises what he or
  she said.
- Repeat back the new statement, client responds again, etc.
- Keep going until the client has achieved insight and self-
  awareness leading to a course of action decision.
- Support the client in acting upon this.

The other is *dialogue*, "interchange and discussion of ideas,
especially when open and frank, as in seeking mutual understanding
or harmony." *Both* parties are active (but courteous) protagonists.
This is a traditional marriage counseling approach:

- One speaks, the other listens carefully.
- The second one repeats back what he or she heard, and responds with clarification, elaboration, rebuttal, revisions,
  and/or proposals.
- Number one does likewise.
- This continues until the two find a mutually acceptable common ground.

There is a third variation, which may be outside the boundaries of

TAP. *Dialectic* (discussed in Chapter 1) is a confrontive version of dialogue in which a position (thesis) is countered with an opposing position (anti-thesis), and hopefully resolved by finding a "third way" which incorporates the best of both (synthesis). Its effectiveness varies among cultures. In New York City, my colleagues would argue thesis-antithesis intensely, hammer out a synthesis, and then go out for a beer together. In Nebraska, with its tradition of courtesy and nonconfrontation, it tends to be counterproductive. In Japan it is downright insulting.

TAP is relevant to a major element of every plan: the question of whom to involve and how. Because it lacks a well-organized framework for getting from here to there, it is rarely the central planning *model*. Elizabeth Bartle (1992), however, has identified circumstances in which it does work:

- When small work groups with similar values are planning to work within a system of varying or dissimilar values. For example, when I work with other radical feminists to plan intervention strategies to combat sexual harassment in the workplace, TAP would seem appropriate . . .
- The interests of participants are not in conflict . . .
- The planners are able to honestly consider the client's experience just as important as their own knowledge base. . . .
- When time is not of the essence. . . . This is a slow process since clients and planners must be open and willing to communicate, adapt, learn from one another and change. For example, using TAP is effective in a feminist collective process with a variety of planners and clients from different backgrounds participating, especially when exploring options other than the status quo is of utmost priority.

Criticisms of Advocacy and Transactive Planning

Critics say that TAP and "pure" GAP applications lack the broad perspective. "Communal, participatory groups can become very self-centered and short-sighted" (Sloter, 1991). They are like a rowboat without a compass. You both steer and propel the boat by hand on short, line-of-sight journeys; that is, by disjointed increments. It's okay for piddling around a pond, but for the ocean and its fast moving currents, you may want a power boat with navigational equipment (such as strategic planning).

TAP (and its cousin, Learning Adaptive) is further criticized for being jumbled and amorphous, with no systematic empirical analysis of either facts or politics. "It is a misty and mutating vision dependent on the changing perceptions of those involved in the dialogue" (Scurfield, 1992).

Practitioners of GAP and TAP have often overestimated their ability to mobilize grassroots people. Professional planners are rarely indigenous to the target subgroup. As outsiders, they often naively misperceive a diverse collection of contiguous individuals in a neighborhood as a homogeneous "community." Is "the black community" in your city monolithic? Do residents of an affluent suburb know, like, and agree with each other? Are there no ego trips or power struggles? The outside planner often ends up allying with, or creating, a power elite within the subgroup, leaving the majority of "members" still unrepresented.

An able and motivated planner may altruistically approach a community with clear notions on what is in its best interest. However, if the local people have a plural-competitive worldview, which is often consistent with their actual life experiences, they will distrust outsiders, particularly self-appointed ones who exhibit ethnocentric ignorance.

Another obstacle is *apathy*, "the general disinterest and political incompetence of many average citizens. . . . These theories do not take into account how the poor often do not have the time or resources to meet and discuss" (Smith, 1991).

All of these pitfalls are beautifully recorded in Lisa Peattie's account (1968) of a group of idealistic young MIT-Harvard planners in 1960s Boston.

It *is* possible for outsiders to help. A major denomination decided to transfer budget control for its Native American mission programs to an intertribal church association. Several national officials met with grassroots Indian leaders. After a day of politely getting nowhere, it was suggested that we break into an "Indian caucus" and a "white caucus." A black official went with the Indians but was courteously invited to "go with the other whites." Then they turned around and asked another official, a lifetime New Yorker with no rural or Native American experience, to join them as a consultant. Why? He was the only one they trusted. A professional CO social worker, he had been relating responsively to them throughout the first day, on their terms and their wave lengths. With his assistance, they settled their own differences, agreed on a plan, and "translated" it into "Anglo" ways of thinking. The conference ended in success.

Another criticism is that advocacy planners may *underestimate* how effectively the establishment puts down unwelcome changes. For starters, look at what happened to GAP. When a new party gained the White House after 1968, it moved quickly to squelch GAP-related activities. It withdrew Community Action Program advocacy funding, cut and then eliminated legal services for the poor, reduced "maximum feasible participation" requirements, re-centralized project grants into block grants to local establishment bodies, and had the IRS run special audits of social agencies that engaged in visible social justice advocacy.

TAP-type projects, on the other hand, have fared better because they are usually low-profile, compartmental activities that are not seen as a political or economic threat to vested interests.

DECENTRALIZED PLANNING

This chapter is not complete without mentioning one more antithesis to centralization, even though it is not directly attached to any participatory method. This is simply to decentralize planning structurally.

There is a continuum from total centralization to anarchy:

- *Imperative.* Central planning and command, as in the military and traditional Communist economies. Obey.
- *Normative.* Central prescriptions are developed for decentralized implementation on a take-it-or-leave-it basis. Needing the benefits, many states, communities, or agencies find this "an offer you can't refuse." For example, project grants and contracts specify objectives and issue an RFP (Request For Proposal) on how you plan to achieve them.
- *Incentive.* Like normative but more permissive, it sets goals and offers rewards to those who plan projects consistent with

the goal. The goal may be relatively specific (a scatter-site housing categorical grant) or broad (an urban development block grant). Subsidies can be direct, as in grants, or indirect, as in free technological support or tax write-offs.

- *Indicative.* Goals and objectives are recommended by a central planning office based on its analyses, but it offers no incentive to the decentralized bodies other than the benefit of taking their wise counsel.
- *Informative.* A central-planning office gathers, analyzes, and distributes intelligence which enables decentralized bodies to make better planning decisions.
- *Laissez faire.* No central intelligence or guidance. Businesses, agencies, and individuals may pursue personal plans on their own without any central informative or indicative input.

The basic rationale for decentralization is that most large organizations or public planning efforts are too complex for full centralization of information, let alone control. Decentralizing means the data for each plan is simpler, cheaper to process, and presumably more accurate. It is quicker to recognize and adapt to change. Decisions are smaller scale, and therefore errors have less impact. Conflicts are resolved at a lower level. It frees up the central planning office for strategic planning and critical major decisions.

The rhetoric says that there will also be more grassroots participation by those affected. My observation has been that this happens much more often within a staff organization than in public planning, where a central elite is merely replaced by an equally unrepresentative local elite.

Decentralization has its limits and liabilities, say other planners. It is more likely to have distortions, to work at cross-purposes with other plans, and to subvert the general mission (if there is one at all). Since decentralization by itself has nothing to say about what methods are used by each plan, there is no assurance that the planning will be more competent, effective, or fair. Indeed, fragmentation guarantees inequitable distribution. A resident of one state may have better highways, education, and health care than an equal citizen in another state.

A SYNTHESIS?

A synthesis of CRAM with its pluralistic antitheses might be a modified strategic planning model, such as *Total Quality Management* (TQM). Keep the central master perspective but (1) widen participation in setting that perspective, and (2) delegate or decentralize specific courses of action (objectives, means, and implementation) to those with a direct knowledge and stake in each subarea as fully as is compatible with the strategic mission. (My experience with TQM projects is that they seem to do the delegating part much better than the upward input.)

REFERENCES

Banfield, E. (1955). "Notes on a conceptual scheme." In Meyerson, M. and Banfield, E., *Politics, planning and the public interest*. New York: Free Press, pp. 303-329.

Bartle, E. (1992). Unpublished paper. University of Nebraska-Omaha.

Cowan, P. (1979). *The future of planning*. London: Heinemann.

Davidoff, P. (1965). "Advocacy and pluralism in planning." *Journal of the American Institute of Planners*, 31, pp. 331-338.

Finks, D. (1984). *The radical vision of Saul Alinsky.* New York: Paulist Press.

Friedman, J. (1973). *Retracking America: A theory of transactive planning*. New York: Doubleday.

Horwitt, S. (1989). *Let them call me rebel: Saul Alinsky—His life and his legacy.* New York: Alfred A. Knopf.

Kahn, S. (1991). *Organizing*. Silver Spring, MD: NASW/1991.

Lindblom, C. (1959). "The science of muddling through." *Public Administration Review*, 19, pp. 79-88.

Lindblom, C. (1968). *The policy making process*. Englewood, NJ: Prentice Hall.

Lindblom, C. (1979). "Still muddling, not yet through." *Public Administration Review*, 39, pp. 517-526.

Peattie, L. (1968). "Reflections on advocacy planning." *Journal of American Institue of Planners*, 34, pp. 80-88.

Rogers, C. (1951). *Client-centered therapy.* Boston: Houghton Mifflin.

Scurfield, G. (1992). Unpublished paper. University of Nebraska-Omaha.

Shaw, G. B. (1948). "Maxims for revolutionaries." Appendix to the play *Man and Superman* in *Nine Plays*. New York: Dodd, Mead, p. 73.

Shaw, G. B. (1906/1977). *The doctor's dilemma*. Harmondsworth, England: Penguin.

Sloter, B. (1991). Unpublished paper. University of Nebraska-Omaha.

Smith, D. (1991). Unpublished paper. University of Nebraska-Omaha.

III. STEP-BY-STEP PROCESS

In Chapter 1, the BASIC model clustered planning processes into six stages, or levels:

1. *Global vision perspective:* the ultimate who, what, where, and why; where you are coming from and where you are going.
2. *Strategic planning:* overview planning, moving from the global perspective to relatively broad middle-range goals.
3. *Tactical planning:* getting down to brass tacks; pinning down the specifics on what you are going to do now and how you plan to do it.
4. *Operational design:* the nitty-gritty; who does what when, step-by-step.
5. *Implementation activity:* doing it and handling what develops.
6. *Evaluation review:* finding out how well you succeeded, and learning things that will improve your future planning.

The three chapters in this section elaborate this model, step by step. Chapter 9 deals with how to clarify global questions, with emphasis on the existing situation, the ultimate goals (desirable situation), and the VIBES that affect them.

Chapter 10 covers both strategic- and tactical-level planning. They are combined in one chapter, because a number of the steps and techniques are parallel in both. Essentially, the global vision is worked down to middle-range goals, and each goal broken into specific objectives and means. Chapter 11 shows how to develop detailed action steps to achieve an objective efficiently.

Together the three chapters offer a method of moving from the ultimate to the immediate.

Chapter 9

Global Vision:
I've Been to the Mountain

I've been to the mountain.

—Martin Luther King, Jr.

Think globally, act locally.

—Lezlie Hartford

"Vision" is an overview perspective. We can't plan without it. How can we get from here to there unless we know what's here and where "there" is? This provides the framework that guides (and evaluates) the specific and practical decisions. It is, for many of us, the most difficult level:

> Few men think in universal terms and vast perspectives. Most of them cling to concrete details and proceed only with difficulty from the specific to the general while the reverse course, starting from powerful principles, appears to them hardly possible at all without previous instruction and training. . . . [They stick to] coastal navigation along clearly discernible shore lines of well-established knowledge, and they do not venture on the high seas of thought and action where the horizons are unlimited. (Zwicky, 1969, p. 3)

WHAT IS THE PLAN ABOUT?

The Source

Although it is theoretically possible to start from the abstract, in most plans someone starts with an *experiential* sense of conditions or circumstances that warrant change (intervention). These are usually problems to be solved or opportunities to be taken.

For practitioners of any field, whether social casework or automobile repair, the first preplanning step is to see a pattern. If the problem comes up only in isolated cases, you treat it individually. If over time you find a recurring pattern in multiple cases, you still treat each case, but you also begin to "think macro." In my field, this is the starting point for most social planning.

Who Plans?

There cannot be a plan without a planner (but not necessarily with a "capital P"). Identify (or create) the planning body and sponsor, such as a government unit, business corporation, service agency, group, or yourself. What are its auspices, authority, acceptability, degree of independence? Who are the individual planners? What do they bring with themselves into the planning process?

What is its fundamental *mission*, both officially and in practice? What *should* its mission be now? Reaffirmed? Clarified? Changed in response to new circumstances or your concerns? Why?

What Are the Boundaries?

What are the direct concerns of this plan: the specific problem or opportunity, relevant conditions and circumstances, the location (geographic, demographic, organizational)? Who are the key actors on whom its success will depend? Who or what are the targets whom it will affect?

What Is Its Context?

Scan the environment within which the planning will occur for elements–political, economic, social, cultural, emotional, physical, and technological–relevant to *this* plan. Even a simple (?) project such as planning for a home of your own involves such real estate and credit market conditions as inflation, home prices in that community, interest rates, down payment requirements, investment return on money being saved for a down-payment, property taxes, and the state of the economy.

Another key context is external ends and interests. How will this plan affect them: positively, negatively, or not at all? First, what are your own interests outside the boundaries of this plan? Second, what are the interests of other actors who can affect the plan? Third, what are the interests of those who will be affected by it, directly or indirectly? These interests may be:

- *Mutually supportive.* Achieving your end enhances the other's interest. Where this is true, there is potential for collaboration and support.
- *Neutral.* Achieving your end has no effect on the other. Generally, in this case you ignore each other.
- *Competitive.* Achieving your end has a negative effect on others' interests. If the impact is modest, it can often be resolved by exchange or compromise. If it is substantial, in order to pursue it, you may need either central authority and control or enough power to win a contention. For instance, environmental planning to save the Everglades and Florida Bay, which calls for restoring water flow that is now pumped away upstream to irrigate sugar, can reasonably expect intense opposition from the sugar growers.

In dealing with external ends and interests, a useful tool is to clarify *actual* versus *perceived* best interests for both yourself and other stakeholders. This can further enhance positives and recast what first appeared to be negatives as actually in a party's *enlightened self-interest*. A husband who has opposed his wife's employment aspirations may come to see material and relationship payoffs for himself in supporting her effort. Some misperceived conflicts may be corrected. Part-time mothering appears to be less in the interests of the children, but in fact there may be a significant qualitative child-rearing gain from a busier but happier mother over a depressed and unfulfilled full-time one.

In addition to determining desirability, it is also *strategically* useful to assess, for bargaining purposes, where both your own and the opponents' interests are *really* intractable, where they are not so conflicting as they seemed at first glance, what is unimportant enough to permit trade-off compromises, and where an apparent obstacle might even be converted into an asset.

WHAT SHOULD BE?

VIBES

First, "get in touch" with your own values, interests, beliefs, ethics, and slants, which will ultimately determine the direction of the plan. They will operate, consciously or unwittingly. We are more in control if we know what they are.

Next, determine how you will treat the VIBES of others. Whose will you take into account: actors who may affect your ability to do the job, those affected directly, the general public? How will you bring them into your planning? (See Chapter 12 on involvement.)

From this review, make your conscious VIBES choices. Based on these, paint the ideal desirable situation, what *should* be, without reference to what is "practical" (that comes later). This guides your sense of purpose and direction. When you encounter rough seas or landslides, it will be your gyroscope ("an apparatus capable of maintaining the same absolute direction in space in spite of movements of the mountings and surrounding parts").

What if you are a "right-brained" thinker, not used to abstract thinking but able to conjure up a vision of the ideal situation? No problem! Make the intuitive leap in your own way, then ask yourself why. That is, analyze it in *retrospect* to be sure it is what you really think. You still end up in the same place: with your head, heart, and gut "in sync."

Long-Range Goals

Within the desirable situation, set broad, ultimate outcome goals. Bicanic (1967) calls it "metaplanning." I call it, "Whatcha wanna be when you grow up?" Branch (1990, pp. 48-49) explains it:

> Whereas planning objectives are specific . . . planning goals are not. Goals identify achievements that are desirable but

cannot be attained for a long time to come. . . . They can be realized gradually by taking advantage of opportunities that arise for incremental advances.

How long is long? Ten years? Twenty years? Fifty years? However far into the future you can project meaningfully. Twenty to thirty years is a normal range. In individual planning with students, I shorten it: "Describe yourself and your work ten years from now as you would like to be." Full achievement is not necessarily expected, given so many uncertainties over such a long period, but it is a real target (not just a utopian fantasy) at which to aim, and in so doing, accomplish more than lower aspirations would have achieved.

How precise should the long-range goal be? Should it be *ambiguous*? The traditional, rationalist answer is no! It should be as clear as possible. Ambiguity is a refuge of politicians and promoters. If you fudge skillfully, you can con the suckers (up to a point) and twist the outcome into a "success" no matter what it is.

On auto trips with my children, I was a congenital explorer of "shortcuts and scenic routes." If it worked, it was a shortcut. If not, I would enthuse, "Wasn't that a beautiful scenic route?" One such "scenic route" turned out to be a potholed road past smelters and slag heaps: I recited Carl Sandburg. (Of course my ungrateful kids soon insisted, gleefully, on more precise goal statements.)

On a more serious level, ambiguous goals can create serious problems of managerial confusion, indecision, even litigation over disputed commitments. At its worst, it can be catastrophic: read Barbara Tuchman's *The March of Folly* (1984), on the British in America and the Americans in Vietnam two centuries apart.

On the other hand. . . Let's play devil's advocate and make a case for "positive ambiguity." Broadly defined goals allow room for refinement, flexibility, contingency adaptations, and feasibility compromises. Nearly everyone will endorse a general goal of adequate income which does not define adequacy or identify the mechanisms by which to achieve it. This is deliberately left ambiguous, for opponents would shoot down anything specific, but they are reluctant to reject openly a motherhood-and-apple-pie goal. Yet it is still relatively clear on some things: that there is a minimum human standard of living, that many people are below it, and that we should do something about it. This umbrella legitimizes a wide variety of incremental and middle-range plans in the public, business, and charitable sectors which chip away at it.

The semi-ambiguous goal lends itself to successive clarifications during the planning process in at least three ways:

- Dialectical argument.
- Heuristic trial and error.
- Decentralized planning, where each "lower" level further clarifies and increases its specificity.

WHAT IS?

Get an overview perspective on the *existing situation*—and the probable future situation given no new intervention. Look at:

- Substantive conditions.
- Procedural circumstances under which things operate.
- Conflicting perceptions about these conditions and circumstances.

From this, draw your conclusions, for planning purposes, about what is.

THE GAP

Compare "what is" with "what should be." The difference is the *gap*. Obviously, any valid planning will be directed to fill this gap in some way, to some degree.

THE CHICKEN OR THE EGG?

Which comes first in our analysis, the chicken (existing situation) or the egg (future desirable condition)? In this day of genetic engineering, the egg comes first. In planning, it logically comes first too. The more nonbounded the thinking is, the better our vision. The existing is measured against it. Martin Luther King Jr.'s, "I have a dream" was an inspired vision of a desirable situation. It guided yet transcended his civil rights strategies, tactical objectives, and means. Without it, his "mountain" might have been a plateau.

> Follow, follow, follow the gleam,
> Standards of worth,
> O'er all the earth,
> Follow, follow, follow the gleam
> To the vision that is the grail.

—Old hymn

On the other hand, the egg is laid by a chicken. Most of my friends start from that direction. First they look at the existing situation, then they ask what should be changed to become a more desirable situation. While nonbounded rationality is theoretically possible, they are usually caught by Burch's Law, with the status quo as the first draft and which controls 85 percent of the final thought.

A realistic compromise is to start wherever we happen to step into the water first. From that particular spot, ascend to the global perspective with thinking as open as we can reasonably muster. It may be a difficult climb at first. We get winded. Our muscles are sore. We are impatient to get back to a level road and make better time. We may turn back before the summit. Don't despair. If you get halfway up, your view, while limited, is wider than if you had stayed in the valley. Next time you can climb to a higher view. It gets easier with practice.

ALWAYS DO GLOBAL THINKING

This process appears to be rather comprehensive, abstract, and difficult. It can be. In many cases it should be. It may be intuitive only. However, more important than the erudition of it is that you are thinking this way at all. Whatever its source, make it explicit to yourself so that you can make conscious choices to affirm or revise it. This puts you back in control of your planning.

It may need only five minutes of quiet thought. I find this sufficient where:

- The planner starts out with a clear sense of direction, which only needs to be recognized and affirmed.
- Other key actors (if any) are on the same wave length.
- The planner is not accountable to others, as in much personal planning.

In other situations, this can be a difficult, time-consuming planning stage. You must know where other actors are coming from. In a national denominational headquarters, it was my diverse constituency. When employed by a corporation and later a university, I had to dope out the authority-sponsor's global thinking. If it is explicit, this may be a quick check. If others' views are covert or, worse, unwitting (as is often the case), we have to investigate further to discover what they really are.

What do you do with this knowledge? That you have to decide. Depending on the situation, a planner might embrace, try to change, loyally obey, or decline to serve. As a national church official, everything I planned was within explicit church pronouncements that coincided with my own beliefs. No sweat.

More often we enter into a limited-liability agreement to do that planning which is mutually acceptable. I was hired by a corporation to help plan its philanthropy and community service. Although my values were altruistic, I narrowed the planning to areas in which the company could "do well by doing good," and further to those "good things" which fitted the vision of each subsidiary's management. In one that had an executive with exceptional vision, we got into creative social change (my personal highest priority): an effective affirmative program in a racially tense city–which won him national recognition. In the other eight subsidiaries, I limited my planning to non-controversial education, health, and cultural areas. The project was a bounded success: each did well within its limits.

REFERENCES

Bicanic, R. (1967). *Problems of planning East and West*. Hague: Mouton.
Branch, M. (1990). *Planning: A universal process*. New York: Praeger.
Tuchman, B. (1984). *The march of folly*. New York: Ballentine.
Zwicky, F. (1969). *Discovery, intervention, and research through the morphological approach*. New York: Macmillan.

Chapter 10

From the General to the Specific

Strategic planning moves from a global foundation to middle-range perspective goals . . . within the scope of the average person's ability to deal with the future.

Bicanic, 1967

STRATEGIC-LEVEL PLANNING

Strategic analysis and planning can be persued through a logical sequence of steps. A six-step sequence is suggested here.

1. Gap Analysis

Strategic analysis begins with a study of the gap between "should be" and "is" identified at the global vision level. This may be initially a broad scan, with a more detailed follow-up in selected areas when the plan moves "down" to specific actions. Gap information falls into five subareas:

- *Substantive* facts about the condition, often called *needs assessment*, including both the condition which is the subject of the plan and other needs and wants which compete for the same resources.
- *Causes* of the condition. This is often called diagnosis, etiology, or epidemiology.
- *Procedural* facts about what can be done. This includes the state of the art, available resources, likely constraints, and the market (competing preferences).

- *Key assumptions* about what is unknown or uncontrollable. This includes both existing elements and expectations about how the future will reflect or differ from the past. Assumptions are updated as new information and experience unfold during the planning.
- *Possible interventions* to eliminate or reduce the gap in light of the causes, procedural facts, and assumptions identified above.

2. Strategic Reduction: Key Result Areas

The planning analysis must be reduced to manageable proportions. This always costs something in accuracy and comprehensiveness. Strategic reduction, typically via a broad overview scan, trims as much fat and bone as possible while preserving the filet.

> Your judgment is necessarily full of arbitrary decisions. . . . You must in any case decide what to notice, what to ignore, and where to stop the calculus of cause and effect. If we make you take these decisions and make these assumptions rationally and explicitly, are they not more likely to be right and will you not be the wiser for knowing more clearly what you have omitted and what you have assumed? (Vickers, 1978, p. 103)

Tenner and DeToro (1992, pp. 118-119) suggest guideline questions for this process:

1. *Have we distinguished the vital few from the trivial many?* Joseph M. Juran believes that a fundamental law of nature dictates that 80 percent of the problems are the result of 20 percent of the causes. . . .
2. *Have we diagnosed the root causes?* Kaoru Ishikawa suggests that the first signs of a problem are its symptoms, not its causes. Actions taken on symptoms cannot be permanently effective . . . .
3. *Do we understand the sources of variation?* . . . . Common causes are inherent within the system . . . and can only be solved by addressing the underlying system.

Pick a "vital few" gap areas in which we want this plan to make a difference, commonly called *key result areas* (KRAs). These are not goals. They are the problem or opportunity areas for which goals (intended results) should be developed. There are two important criteria for prioritizing them.

One is *whose interests?* Most plans involve competing interests. A KRA gives preference to some over others. One factor in ranking KRAs is one's earlier VIBES decision about their relative priority. (See Chapters 2 and 9.)

The other is *state of need.* Which needs/wants are greatest, taking into account such factors as the quantity of a need, its intensity, and consequences of not meeting it? (See Chapter 13.)

Rate possible KRAs in priority categories, such as essential, high, moderate, low. Eliminate the low-priority ones. Normally relegate the moderate ones to a back burner for possible future consideration. Put essential and high ones on a "short list" from which you will then select the one (or more) KRA which this plan will address.

3. Candidate Goals

Within the KRA, elaborate alternative goals that meet the following tests:

- An *end result* which closes all or part of the gap within that KRA.
- *Middle range*, broad yet one which you really aim to achieve over time.
- *Clearly enough* stated to tell whether, and when, you achieve it.

Routinely add, for comparison in the desirability review, the *default alternative of no intervention.* Sometimes not acting may promise a better outcome. The hospice movement offers an alternative to "heroic" treatment plans for terminally ill persons. Classical economic theory opposes any planning of the economy in favor of the "natural law" of unrestricted market competition (laissez faire).

4. Desirability Review

Do a desirability-undesirability review of each candidate, and compare the results to help guide which you select to go forward.

Some general criteria to consider in reviewing and selecting for desirability include:

- *Potential effectiveness:* its contribution to closing the gap if achieved.
- *Urgency.* What are the consequences of deferring it?
- *Horizontal compatibility* with your other ends and interests. Does it enhance them, subvert them, or have no effect? These may include specific programs and plans as well as intangibles such as quality of life, relationships, esteem, and integrity.
- *Value-ethics-ideology compatibility.*
- *Spillover* effects on others. Positive side effects increase overall desirability; bad ones may negate an otherwise good plan.
- *Acceptability* to targets and others affected by the plan.
- *Opportunity cost:* the net benefit compared to what could have been done instead with the same resources.

Applying this to a particular plan, you may want to be more specific. For instance, in personal career planning, "contribution to closing the gap" might, depending on the KRA, be specified as professional growth and development, satisfaction, income, or security. "Horizontal compatibility" might become effect on family life.

If there are many candidate goals, try a mixed-scanning approach, like running the sand of a pebbly beach through a series of sieves. The large hole sieve catches out the big stones and lets the rest through; the next sieve screens out middle-sized gravel, and so on, until the final sieve, that passes only the finest sand.

First, eliminate those goals which have unacceptable negatives in such areas as horizontal compatibility, ethics, or harmful side effects. Second, scratch those whose level of contribution is too low to be worth pursuing. Then do a final, careful review of the not-bad survivors to pick the few candidate goals that are worthwhile enough to warrant a serious feasibility review.

5. Feasibility Review

Two clergymen were walking to the station. The first said, "Hurry, or we'll miss the train." The second replied confidently,

"According to my watch there is plenty of time, and I have complete faith in it." They slowed down–and arrived to find the train gone. "You see," said the first, "faith by itself without good works is dead."

In planning, desirability without good works is dead. The second essential review is feasibility: *can it be done?* Among feasibility factors to look at are:

- Ability to generate *specific objectives.*
- Availability of *resources.*
- *Affordability* of costs.
- Sufficient *flexibility* to adjust to contingencies.
- Enough *time* available to carry it out.

Earlier, at the global vision level, only desirability was considered. Later, at the objective-means tactical plan level, the accent was heavily on practical feasibility. At this strategic stage, desirability is dominant, but feasibility has veto power. A negative scan may be appropriate. Eliminate those which cannot generate potentially doable specific objectives or appear to have little or no chance of meeting the other criteria.

What if the answer is an inconclusive "maybe"? This is a judgment call. Incrementalists eliminate everything that isn't a "sure thing." I lean the other way: keep alive at this stage any goal that isn't clearly out of the question. It is amazing how often I have found a way to do something which my colleagues would have written off. Henry Ford said, "Whether you think you can or think you can't, you're right!"

6. The Final Goal

We have reduced our candidate goals to a short list. We have judged each to be both desirable and feasible. There may not be a large difference among them. Yet we don't have the resources to do them all, at least not all at once.

There is no simple formula for choosing the best goal from among them. Among the possible approaches:

- The most *desirable.*
- The apparently most *feasible.*

- An optimum *compromise* of desirability with achievability. Chapter 19 lays out a formal quantitative method for doing this, with the aid of a few "stochastic" guesses where data is insufficient. Such a choice may also be made intuitively, based on accumulated insight and experience.
- *Paired comparisons*. This works like a demolition derby. Take any two and compare them. Keep the better, eliminate the lesser. Pair any two more and eliminate the lesser. Keep going until there is only one left running. The formal logic: if A is better than B, then it is also better than everything that B can beat.

Multiple Goals?

The simplest model assumes that the plan will have a single goal at the strategic level. This is not always the case. There are two excellent reasons to have multiple goals.

One is necessity. Sometimes a set of goals are symbiotic ("the living together of two distinct organisms in close association or union when this is advantageous or necessary to both"). You can't solve unemployment with a worker-training goal if the jobs aren't there, nor can you create new jobs through economic development if the skilled workers aren't available. The only sound way to go is to do both concurrently in a coordinated dual plan.

When I was in the Labor Department, Louis Sullivan's Opportunities Industrial Corporation in inner-city Philadelphia was greatly outperforming our own Manpower Development and Training Act programs. I was assigned to find out why. We had a single goal—training—after which the worker looked for a job. Our employment success rate was a creditable 50 percent. Sullivan had two goals. One was training. The other was placement. OIC canvassed local employers about jobs they needed to fill and the skills required, and trained workers for those specific jobs. Employers themselves participated in the training. Not surprisingly, OIC's employment rate was close to 100 percent.

The other good reason for multiple goals is capacity. If you have enough resources to pursue several separately, there is no reason not to pursue as many different goals as you can handle at one time. I can pursue career, family, health, and recreation goals concurrently (with a bit of scheduling, of course).

If you do have multiple goals, consider developing and delegating them as separate subplans within a coordinating master strategy umbrella.

TACTICAL-LEVEL PLANNING

A man of words and not of deeds,
Is like a garden full of weeds.

—Benjamin Franklin

Specific means "definite, precise, having a limited application." This is the stage of moving from broad goals to concrete here-and-now objects and means. A six-step sequence for the process is offered below.

1. Decomposition

Break down the goal into manageable components which can be readily grasped and acted upon.

2. Candidate Objectives

Identify alternative objectives that meet *all* of the following criteria. Drop or modify those which do not.

- Contributes to achievement of the goal, directly or as a stepping stone.
- Is a result (end), not an activity (means).
- Is specific and concrete.
- Is time limited, with a due date.
- Is measurable, quantitatively where possible, so that you can tell whether, when, and how well it has been achieved.

Candidate objectives can be:
- *Mutually exclusive.* If so, you must choose one against the other.

- *Sequential.* A stepping-stone objective may not directly achieve a piece of the goal but is necessary in order to achieve subsequent objectives which will. Let's say one's goal is a master's thesis. Stepping-stone objectives (prerequisites) may be completion of courses in (1) statistics, (2) basic research methods, and (3) advanced research methods.
- *Interdependent.* These should be scheduled together.
- *Separate and unrelated.* These can be scheduled sequentially in order of priority or, as resources permit, concurrently.

3. Candidate Tactical Plans

Strategy is the framework within which tactical moves are made. Strategy comes first. Tactics implement strategies.

—Steiner, 1979

"Love and marriage, love and marriage/Go together like a horse and carriage." A *tactical plan* is a course of action that consists of *both the objective and the means by which it will be pursued.* If you want the end ("love"), it must be combined with an effective means ("marriage"): "Dad was told by Mother/You can't have one without the other."

There is more than one way to skin a cat. The same objective may be accomplished through more than one means. At one time I traveled frequently from New York to Washington. The objective was always the same, but I had a choice between three means: drive, fly the shuttle, ride AMTRAK. These means were significantly different in time, cost, stress, convenience, reliability, and side effects.

For each candidate objective, identify the different possible means. Each separate objective-means combination is an alternative tactical plan.

There is a dialectic here. CRAM chooses the objective first. Only then, having set the course, does it address and select possible means to get there. Why waste your time checking out means for objectives you haven't chosen?

Disjointed incrementalism does it the other way around. First find out what resources are available to you. Then consider only objectives which are within that reach. Why waste your time on pie in the sky?

In the BASIC model synthesis, we go back and forth freely between objectives and means all along the way.

4. Assessment of Tactical Plans

Desirability factors for tactical plans are a more concrete version of those spelled out for goals: contribution toward reaching the goal, urgency, horizontal compatibility, ethics, side effects, and acceptability.

Feasibility receives careful attention at the tactical level. Some of the factors are:

- *Do-ability:* a mix of two related factors: (1) the state of the art—how successful can anyone be?; and (2) your capability under actual circumstances.
- *Design:* ability to succeed if it is carried out as planned.
- Availability and affordability of *resources* needed to do it.
- *Support of superiors* (bosses, funders, regulators).
- Motivation and commitment of staff and other *implementers.*
- Acceptability to *target* groups, consumers, other stakeholders.

A simple chart can be used to assess each candidate tactical plan. In the chart below, A, B, and C are alternative agency expansion tactical plans. This chart lists six feasibility factors, giving each a score of 4 to 0 on the standard A to F grade-point system. Such insightful "rough and ready" ratings do not use precise, consistent interval numbers and therefore cannot be manipulated to provide valid statistical data. (See Chapter 15.) However, it does help us clarify our thinking.

	A	B	C
Do-ability	4	3	3
Design	4	3	3
Resources	3	4	2
Superiors	2	4	2

	A	B	C
Implementers	3	4	2
Targets	4	2	3

Eyeballing the chart, we decide to drop C because it grades quite a bit lower than the other two. That's the easy part.

A and B have similar numbers overall. Although it gives us no "answer," the chart clarifies the strengths and weakness of A and B, enabling a given planner to make a decision based on his or her view of what feasibility factors are most important. An "optimizing" professional may prefer A because it is the technically best plan and most responsive to clients (targets). A satisficing bureaucrat, on the other hand, may choose B, which has a "good enough" design and, more important to him, maximum support from those who matter.

We can further quantify our judgments by giving a relative importance weight (say, 1 to 4) to each of the feasibility factors. Multiply each number on the above chart by the item's importance number to get a weighted score. (See section on "Utility" in Chapter 18.) If "target" is given an importance of 4, the weighted score of A on this measure is 16 (4 $\times$ 4). If its importance is 2, the weighted score is 8 (4 $\times$ 2). Feel free to do such weighting and even to add up the results to a total score for each tactical plan if it helps you, so long as you don't forget that the numbers are neither more nor less than a reflection of your own values and judgments.

Another popular framework, TWOS (Threats, Weaknesses, Opportunities, Strengths; alias SWOT or WOTS), helps to identify specific positive and negative feasibility factors. List your best estimate of reality factors in each box.

	FUTURE		PRESENT	
	Internal	External	Internal	External
OBSTACLES	Threats		Weaknesses	
ASSETS	Opportunities		Strengths	

- *Threats* are potential obstacles, such as opposition or a budget cuts.
- *Weaknesses* are existing deficiencies in power, resources, and staff, as well as blockages and organizational constraints. An illustration of blockage was my "bad old dean" who suffered from lack of integrity, limited vision, and his superiors' distrust. Any innovative plan was much more difficult through this bottleneck than under his successor, a clear-eyed, caring person with savvy and skills, who changed the Dean's Office into a "strength."
- *Opportunities* are potentials that can enhance the strengths and shore up the weaknesses. Positive contingencies may be anticipated, such as the chance of a special grant or budget increase.
- *Strengths* are existing resources, whatever can be used toward achieving one's ends: competence and expertise, creative thinking, organization, motivation, budget, time, power. It includes that which is within your direct control plus what you can count on from others.

I have found it useful to further break down TWOS, into internal and external threats, weaknesses, opportunity and strengths.

5. Final Selection

Eliminate any tactical plan that is:

- *Unacceptable:* has significant undesirable qualities, including ethics.
- *Infeasible:* is unlikely to succeed.
- *A net loss:* costs more than its benefits.

You now have only acceptable objective-means combinations (tactical plans). Use some kind of comparative approach which takes into account desirability, feasibility, *and* cost benefit. (See Chapter 18.) If you use a quantified method, test the apparent best choice against your common sense, intuition, and the consensus of key actors. If they all coincide, go with it. If not, better chew on it some more.

When you select one, don't necessarily throw the others away. You may want to come back to some of them in one of three ways.

One way is to *defer* them. In the case of stepping-stone objectives, put them into a logical time sequence.

If they are parallel to the selected one, *queue* them up to be pursued when resources become available. My program had parallel objectives of hiring a professor in each of three subject areas, but only one opening. We achieved one objective that year, and the other two as positions became available later.

A second way is to keep the runner-up "vice plan" (alias Plan B) as a *contingency*. A variation of this is the unburnt bridge: carrying out one objective in a way that does not close the door on alternative objectives. A student choosing between a master's and a doctoral program may pursue a master's which provides professional credentials in itself and also offers credits that can be applied to a later doctorate.

A *concurrent* approach is to act simultaneously on a cluster of objectives and means: "moving ahead with everything and everybody, all together and all at once, toward a specific goal" (Schriever, 1958). This may require an old-fashioned master plan in which the whole network is diagrammed and delegated with detailed lines of support, accountability, and coordination drawn. This is standard for large-scale plans, crisis-disaster responses, and some personal planning (such as scheduling four different courses per semester).

6. Evaluation

After the specific objective has been selected but before implementation, develop an evaluation design to measure how well we succeed. Doesn't evaluation come at the end? Then why must we design it before we act? Two reasons.

First, it is necessary for the evaluation itself. Before-and-after comparisons are an almost universal evaluation tool. Since you can't collect baseline data after you have intervened, you have to know, before you start, what you will need.

Second, it is part of pinning down the goals and objectives. The evaluation design is the final test of the soundness and clarity of your objective. If you can't define it sufficiently to evaluate, it is probably also too vague to carry out efficiently.

REFERENCES

Bicanic, R. (1967). *Problems of planning East and West*. Hague: Mouton.

Schriever, B. (1958). *The USAF report on the ballistic missile*.

Steiner, G. (1979). *Strategic planning*. New York: Free Press.

Tenner, A. and DeToro, I. (1992). *Total quality management*. Reading, MA: Addison-Wesley.

Vickers, G. (1978). *Value systems and social progress*. Baltimore: Penguin.

Chapter 11

Blueprint for Action: Project Management

Success is most likely to occur when know-how is teamed with know-when.

—Anon.

PROJECT MANAGEMENT AND "PERT"

A project is a unique piece of work having a finite life and producing an identifiable product or achieving a specific aim on time and within specified resource limits.

—Canadian Government

Project management is a general term for laying out a comprehensive operational plan to achieve a specified objective, step-by-step. It uses linear programming and networking.

Origins

It all began with industrial engineering techniques, such as Henry Ford's assembly line, where each work station did a specific job in a linear order. The product moved straight down the line. There were sublines which put together a fender or a door, and these fed like tributaries into the mainstream assembly line at just the point where they were needed. Other techniques include flow charts, process charts, and crew balance studies.

In the late 1950s, two groups developed computerized programs to expand the assembly-line concept to an elaborate network of lines (renamed "paths") for implementing every activity of a plan. One was the Critical Path Method (CPM) developed at Dupont. The other was the Program Evaluation and Review Technique (PERT) developed to shorten the time required to build the first nuclear submarine. The two merged into one stream (with a few side eddies), using both names more or less interchangeably. Incremental variations have spun off, often sprouting their own names, notably Precedence Diagraming Method (PDM). A variety of computer programs are available at all levels from a Pentagon supercomputer to a PC.

The convention used in this chapter is a version of PDM presented by John Mulvaney in *Analysis Bar Charting—As Easy As ABC* (1975). However, I will refer to the process by the common generic names, *PERT* and *Project Management*.

If you are not already expert, learn first to apply PERT at a simple manual level, using hands, head, and index cards. Once clear and comfortable with the straightforward logic of it, you can make better use of the computerized versions. If you start directly with a complex computer program, you may end up following the manual by blind rote without the understanding to adapt it more effectively to your particular project.

What It Is

After the specific "objective-means combination" has been selected, PERT breaks it down into a detailed schedule of bite-size activities, arranged in coordinated sequences. It follows a closed mechanical system model which assumes that the short-term future is fixed and predictable. In practice, however, good project managers regularly adjust to contingencies.

PERT anticipates everything that must be done, the resources needed, and the order in which it should be carried out. It looks for the shortest, most efficient route.

The general process:

1. Define a clear, unequivocal *finish point* (concrete objective).
2. Identify the precise *starting point* (here and now).

3. Develop a *project design*. Identify all tasks which need to be accomplished to reach the finish line. Order them into *steps* on a *path*. Paths are laid out in sequence, with each earlier step a prerequisite for the ones that follow. Steps which are independent of each other proceed down *parallel* paths. Paths may divide at one point and converge at another.
4. *Schedule* the project, taking into account activities for each step, the time needed to complete them, and the cumulative time required to complete the whole path.
5. *Control* the project, "seeing that the tasks are executed according to the project plan and making the necessary decisions and adjustments when deviations occur" (Jackman, 1990, p. 27).

JOBS AND PATHS

Jobs

Each step in a PERT chart is a *job* (task) which consists of a specific *end* to be achieved and the *activity* to accomplish it. Jobs are commonly designated by numbers or letters, with an attached key that identifies the job each represents. (Because you use numbers for time periods, labeling jobs with letters is visually less confusing on a manual PERT.)

The original CPM model had beads on a string to denote *events* (completion points of jobs). The activity to complete an event is shown as a line or arrow:

Start ⟶ A ⟶ B ⟶ C ⟶ Finish

The model used in this chapter looks like an old tenement "Pullman apartment," where the rooms were in a line without hallways. You had to go through the living room to the kitchen and thence through the first bedroom to get to the second bedroom. Each job is a box that you must pass through to get to the next. The right end of the box ($\|$) is the finish of the job (the event). The left end of the box is the start of activity on the job. The space between left and right is the activity.

Start ⊣ ☐ A ☐⊢ ☐ B ☐⊢ ☐ C ☐⊢ Finish

Paths

A path is one *sequence of jobs* from start to finish, each a prerequisite for the next. There may be any number of paths.

As an illustration, let's run through an abridged version of the PERT design to earn a degree in my program, including prerequisites and sequences. The jobs are individual courses.

A. Human behavior
B. General practice (prerequisite: A)
C. Individual counseling (pre: B)
D. Individual therapy (pre: C)
E. Group therapy (pre: D)
F. Family therapy (pre: D)
G. Policy analysis
H. Community organization (pre: B and G)
 I. Supervision (pre: C and H)
J. Social change (pre: H)
K. Statistics
L. Basic research methods (pre: K)
M. Advanced research methods (pre: L)
N. Research project (pre: M)

Parallel paths are sequences that do not overlap and therefore can be done at the same time. Below, the therapy path is separate from the research path, but both are required for the degree (finish):

```
         ┌ B- C- D- E-┐
Start ──┤            ├─ Finish
         └ K- L- M- N-┘
```

Split paths have common beginnings but later diverge into parallel paths. Below, after the introductory common course (B), the practice track splits into micro and macro practice paths:

```
              ┌ C- D- E-┐
Start - B ──┤          ├- Finish
              └ H- J ───┘
```

Parallel paths may merge at a later point into a path whose tasks have multiple pre-requisites. Below, supervision (I) requires prior training in both micro and macro practice skills:

Start – B ⌈ C ⌉ I – Finish
       ⌊ H ⌋

The whole chart looks like this:

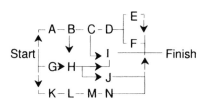

This chart has eight paths: ABCDE, ABCDF, ABCI, ABHI, ABHJ, GHI, GHJ, KLMN.

The Backward Pass

The *logic* of PERT is deductive from the objective. This means starting at the finish and *working backward*.

In the above illustration, the objective (finish) is an MSW degree. What do you have to have to get there? Answer: competence in several parallel areas–therapy, macro practice, supervision, and research.

Let's do a backward pass on therapy. To be qualified, you need individual, group, and family therapy skills. What do you need to be ready for group and family therapy (E & F)? Individual therapy skills (D). What do you need to be prepared to study individual therapy? General counseling skills (C). What do you need for that? Basics skills such as problem solving and creative listening (B). What foundation do you need for basic skills? Human behavior (A).

Now follow the research path back. You need an independent research project (N) to graduate. To design and carry it out, you need to know advanced research methods (M). To understand advanced research methods, you must already know basic research methods (L). That research course assumes a knowledge of basic statistics (K).

Although this logic and process is simple enough, it runs counter to our normal instinct to think and act forward from beginning to end. Many people find it difficult to reverse their thinking for

PERT's backward pass even though it makes sense to do so. Yet, programming forward almost guarantees that we will overlook a step somewhere, add another which is not necessary, and incur delays due to errors in sequence.

In my Labor Department planning, veteran bureaucrats habitually implemented in a certain methodical step-by-step way. In the new poverty-youth training project, they moved into a new territory of timing, clients, and type of grantee agency—but did their standard forward pass, which slowed our "crash program" to a walk and discouraged local grantee response. The task had to be shifted to "newcomer" planners, who did a backward pass specifically related to this program's objectives and circumstances. Unnecessary steps did not intrude. Activities new to the Department were added. The result: a faster, more effective process.

Perhaps there is a comfortable compromise with the "backwards" problem. I allowed beginning students or staff to start out by identifying steps "any which way" and to put them into paths by standard forward thinking. They did pretty well, coming up with a majority of the needed steps, and avoided getting bogged down in laboriously unfamiliar deduction.

With a concrete first draft (however imperfect), they were then able to do the rigorous backward review and revision rather comfortably. They discovered and added overlooked steps. They cut unnecessary steps. They moved some steps from one sequence into a parallel path, and others the reverse. The bottom line: effective backward logic without agony.

Once designed, the implementation of a PERT is comfortably forward-pass (in which my veteran Labor Department colleagues proved, not surprisingly, to be more expert than the newcomers).

Pitfalls

The most common problems associated with PERTing are:

- *Vague objective.* PERT requires a clearly defined finish.
- *Unstructured approach.* If you plunge immediately into the detailed level of jobs and paths without first developing a broad overview-framework, you will probably become hope-

lessly scattered and disorganized, especially in the areas which require coordination (interpath connections).

- *Too much detail and data.* Computer capabilities can seduce you into "analytical overkill," losing your perspective in the mass of detail. A related pitfall is overprescribing actions and procedures so exhaustively that they stifle staff initiative, creativity, and satisfaction. If a work team has poured 100 foundations, it does not need a twenty-box sequence on how to do it. One box with clear specification of end-line standards will do. Moreover, the greater the detail, the less flexibility the implementer has to handle small contingencies.
- *Not enough detail* to identify and coordinate all needed inputs on schedule. If you delegate too much autonomy and self-direction to implementers, they may stray off course relative to the rest of the convoy.
- *Normal errors.* No matter how conscientiously you do a PERT, you deserve a medal if you do not miss or misplace a step somewhere. Frequently overlooked by persons with limited administrative experience are the many administrative, board, regulatory, agency, and political clearances required.

MULTISTAGE PERTING

Multistage PERTing can minimize the unstructured, too-much, and not-enough pitfalls above. It enables you to keep overall perspective and to vary the amount of detail according to the needs of each job.

First Run: Milestone PERT

Don't do the whole PERT in one fell swoop. Not all steps are created equal. As we move along the path, some steps are designated as milestones ("a significant event marking a stage in a journey"). Block out a first run in broad strokes covering a dozen or so key milestones on a few "mainline" paths. These are the most important hurdles to cross, often a culmination of a series of steps. Jobs at intersections where paths split or merge are often milestone points for integrating the entire chart. The *milestone PERT* becomes the skeleton on which the rest of the project's anatomy is hung.

When the full PERT has been developed, these milestones will be checkpoints to monitor progress. In one project to develop a new group home, the milestones included: proposal approved by board, program developed, site found, funding assured, facility bought, facility remodeled and furnished, staff qualifications and training needs determined, staff hired, staff training completed, and clients in residence.

Second Run: Regular PERT

This is elaborated from the milestone PERT. Hal Jackman (1990) calls this process *Work Breakdown Structure:* "WBS subdivides the various project tasks into smaller units until they are manageable activities."

As noted, this is a logical sequence of steps in multiple paths. If done manually, limit the number of jobs to what you can handle without feeling overwhelmed. If the number gets too large, use the third run option below to bring it back down to size. There is no a priori limit on a computerized PERT. The Polaris project had many thousands of steps.

Third Run: SubPERTs

If the regular PERT gets too complicated, you may cluster a group of jobs into one step, asterisk it, and attach a "subPERT." That single *cluster step* becomes a mini-PERT in itself, with a start, a finish, and any number of intermediate steps. The job time of the cluster step is, of course, the project time of its subPERT.

In three kinds of circumstances, this optional third run probably ought to be standard:

- A manual PERT that is more complex than one hand-drawn chart can handle.
- SubPERTing is delegated to units or individuals experienced in the job. Sometimes this is done in a high-structure pattern such as MBO (Management by Objective). Others use a participatory approach such as TQM.

• Mixed-competence staffing. You may want to use a broader PERT for the competent majority, yet give detailed guidance on certain jobs performed by less-qualified workers. To achieve an assembled new bicycle, just give my handy son the box and say you want the bike–but you'll have to give me a detailed subPERT for every nut and bolt.

HOW DETAILED?

Classical PERT, developed in a comprehensive planning context, is exhaustive. For mere mortals, however, I recommend the *Law of Parsimony*: don't do more than you need.

Jackman (1990) is on the right track with his WBS. Break it down as far as is necessary to make the job units manageable. No more. No less. Increase the level of detail to the extent that:

• Implementers are newer to tasks and less able or reliable.
• Interfaces are more numerous and complex.
• Precise specifications and coordination are required. Constructing a spaceship requires a tighter PERT than building a shed.
• Tasks are more elaborate and difficult.
• Resources are tight and rationed.

Reduce the detail to the extent that:

• Reliable old pros are doing it.
• The tasks are routine and repetitive.
• The paths are few and simple.

Be practical. Stay within your limits. Better a modest car on the road than a high-performance model in the showroom. Especially in manual PERTs, there is a point of diminishing returns, beyond which the benefit of refinements is outweighed by becoming too complicated. Further, no matter how good you are at PERTing, don't go beyond what you will actually use. Remember the old Army mess hall motto, "Take all you want, but eat all you take."

MANUAL SORTING

Don't try to draft a PERT on a piece of paper. You will cross out, add, and move jobs and paths so often that it will soon become illegible, or you will be spending all your time recopying the chart over and over. "The only way to go" is a separate card for each job. Spread them out on the conference table, the kitchen table, or the rug. Put them together, look the pattern over, and rearrange to your heart's content. (A good computer program lets you do the same thing faster and better, of course.)

Two heads are better than one. Dialogue (or trialogue?) spots things that one alone may miss. A team is nice. Everyone feeds in one's ideas, then someone lays it out and they discuss and debate, propose, play devil's advocate, and so forth until they are satisfied they have missed nothing important.

"Lay persons" make excellent second heads. If you explain what you are about, a spouse or friend sees with fresh eyes things which you were too close to the trees to notice. (Note: this is true at other planning stages too.)

Review and revise to increase efficiency and/or reduce the project time. First, eliminate any step that is expendable. Second, is each apparent prerequisite really "pre"? If not, move it to a parallel path, thereby increasing flexibility for juggling the schedule of assignments. When you have completed the arranging, draw the chart. Later, at the scheduling stage, you will elaborate it further.

TIME AND RESOURCES FOR EACH STEP

Identify in advance the resources needed for each job and the time required to accomplish it. An accurate estimate avoids waste, delays, and failures.

Involving Key Actors

To get reliable estimates of job requirements, go to the people who know. Experienced staff are in the best position to estimate what is needed. A manager—and even more, an outside planner may be vague and overoptimistic. Make sure the "doers" understand clearly what is wanted, then listen.

Of course, you have to evaluate their reliability. In my national church office, staff were congenitally optimistic, so I often increased their estimates of time and resources needed. In the Labor Department, cautious overestimates were the norm, so I tightened the schedule. In a well-run direct service agency, I found the staff to be both honest and knowledgeable in estimates, so I went with what they recommended. In all three cases, staff input contributed to my scheduling.

Providers of resources are another set of key actors. To plan realistically, you must have a good reading on what you will have to work with. What are they *able* to provide? What is the competition for those resources? What are they *willing* to provide? Are they rigid or open to rational persuasion? Will they be flexible in responding to unexpected contingencies? Are there alternative or supplementary sources you've not considered?

In addition to the information, such involvement offers a valuable second dividend. People who give you commitments on resources and time lines "own" them and are more highly motivated to fulfill them than those who just obey orders. "Dictated task completion is the surest way to failure I know. Conversely, any subordinate who accepts a deadline that he or she cannot commit to is a loser" (Shelmerdine, 1989, p.17).

A key factor in a successful PERT is your boss, who must:

- Understand planning in general, and PERT in particular.
- Respect and appreciate it.
- Make commitments to it.
- Honor commitments.

A colleague of mine was the ablest member of a university urban planning center headed by a loose administrator. She obtained many grant projects for which she developed PERTs. All were signed off by the boss–who then proceeded to ignore his commitments. He "borrowed" already-scheduled project staff. He periodically even took her off the project to pull colleagues' chestnuts out of the fire. Nevertheless, like the Hebrews under Pharaoh, she was held strictly accountable for the success or failure of her "bricks without straw" projects.

So . . . don't PERT with imPERTinent bosses. PERT is premised on the assumption that the future (as it affects the project) is predictable and assured. In an arbitrary and capricious setting, a politicized one, or just an incompetent one, you simply can't assume that. However, in such a setting, half a loaf may still be possible. You can quietly PERT your own piece of the action, taking into account the administrative deficiencies of a boss. With personal clarity about the situation, I have been able to bring a shortsighted boss along pretty well, one step at a time.

Job Resources

For each job, identify every activity required to accomplish it. For each activity, identify every resource needed, including:

- Person hours or days. Specifically, what person(s)?
- Nonpersonnel resources: equipment, materials, space, computer time, software, etc.
- Approvals and authorizations.

Confirm the availability of needed resources. First, do they exist at all? Second, are they available to your project? Third, are they affordable?

What is already committed and unavailable because of mandated programs or other established priorities? If 80 percent of staff workload is contractually dictated or repetitive, only 20 percent at most is available for special PERT jobs unless released from other assigned duties. (My university and church employers used an alternative: unpaid overload.)

Are the resources certain? What is the competition for those resources? Who/what are your competitors for them? Can you get more resources and speed up the project? Can you live with lower resources if you stretch it out longer? Where the resources are insufficient for the job as planned, are there substitute means for which resources are available? How much clout do you have to obtain (and keep!) the resources needed? To complete a reliable PERT design, these uncertainties must be resolved.

If what is available is inadequate, adjust to it. In a minor case, you can work this out intrajob. If it is more serious, it may be necessary to loop back and revise the objective downward. One of the key benefits of PERT is this: by discovering what is not feasible *before* you start, you avoid coming a cropper later.

Job Time

Now you know the jobs, their activities, the resources available, and the hours of staff time required. Next, estimate how many real workdays or weeks the project will require. Abstract statistical analyses are sometimes off base (usually underestimating time needed) because they have failed to take into account "nonproductive" time.

Coffee breaks, chatting, and other "nonproductive" work time, be they good or bad, occupy one-eighth of working hours. Vacation, sick leave and holidays, account for another one-eighth. Add to these normal staff meetings, supervisory conferences, travel and training, plus all the staffing problems identified earlier. Many PERTers discount working hours by 25 percent or more.

You may occasionally vary productivity estimates according to the individuals who are doing that job. When I was director of an academic program, my energetic secretary, a Phi Beta Kappa college graduate, was an "up." For job time estimates, I projected her output as double a normal day's work. In the government, I was assigned a secretary who was just as reliably certain to do a normal half-day load each day (because she "got a load on" at lunch).

When would you want to be this precise? Not on a large project where variations will presumably average out. Not where you have covered this sort of contingency with a built-in tolerance reserve. On the other hand, at the small end of the scale, "where two or three are gathered together," you cannot hope for reliable estimates without individualizing productivity.

Another key factor is *lead time*. If agency board clearance is possible only on first Wednesdays, schedule a clearance date and work your steps back from there (e.g., materials must be mailed at least a week in advance) to figure minimum lead time. If you need printing, what is the delivery or turnaround time? This in turn sets up a deadline for finished copy. Reserving a training site and date may require less work but more lead time than preparing the training content itself. In calculating lead time, don't forget the delays around vacation and holiday periods.

High, Medium, or Low Estimates?

Traditional CPM (Critical Path Method) scheduling is a fixed time based on the implicit assumption of certainty. (Best guess is treated as fact.)

The "official" PERT variation takes uncertainty into account with three time estimates. We can illustrate it with time estimates for completing my department's 42-credit advanced program. The maximum load is a very heavy 15 in fall and spring, 12 in summer. The minimum is 6 each in spring and fall and 0 in summer.

- *Optimistic*, minimum time: 12 months (15/15/12).
- *Pessimistic,* maximum time: 41 months (6/6/0, 6/6/0, 6/6/0, 6).
- *Middle*, average circumstances. In our case, we have two middle choices. For part-time students with heavy outside responsibilities, 29 months (6/6/6, 6/6/6, 6); for full-time students, 21 months (9/9/6, 9/9).

  Use the *optimistic time* when:
- There is external time pressure. I was hired to rebuild a program from scratch to keep it from closing. Given all that needed to be accomplished, a middle-time estimate would be two to three years. Our ultimatum: one year or kaput! A middle course was out of the question.
- You have meticulously accurate calculations and maximum control over key variables or excess capability to throw in if necessary.
- You seek stretch, to push yourself and staff to higher performance.

Optimism has its pitfalls. A project manager scheduled the input of others based on her own high level of productivity, which they did not share. It led to high-stress deadline crises. I suggested she double the work times for tasks her colleagues performed. The next project was still tight, but manageable.

The optimistic time frame is also vulnerable to unpredictable events, such as a blizzard, illness, family crises, or equipment breakdown. Every contingency is a potential crisis.

Use the *pessimistic* time when security is more important than time or efficiency:

- You work in a negative-evaluation system, common in large bureaucracies and poorly managed programs of any size. There is no reward for high performance, but there are sanctions for missing a deadline. On some contracts, there is a financial penalty for each day beyond the promised date. A prudent planner covers oneself by being deliberately pessimistic.
- You want to look good by delivering above expectations.
- There is no urgent deadline. Therefore, efficient time is unimportant.
- High uncertainty. A Murphy's Law inflator may be prudent in your time estimates.

A pitfall of this is that a pessimistic schedule may become a self-fulfilling prophecy.

Unless you have a reason to select high or low expectations, a realistic middle ground with some flexibility for contingency is usually best. In a good organization, you will be rewarded for your efficiency and exonerated for circumstances which neither you nor your boss (who presumably approved the plan) could foresee.

Charting Job Time

Put the job time (hours, days, or weeks) into each box. A simple conventional format:

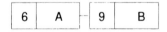

SCHEDULING PROJECT TIMES

The jobs are now set in their paths with job times assigned. Next we do a simple *forward pass* to determine the *early times* of each job and path. Put the early times above the box.

On the illustration below, the earliest possible start time for the first job on each path (A and F) is 0. Job A takes six days, so its earliest finish time is 6. This in turn becomes the earliest starting time for B, the next job on that path. When two or more paths merge, the earliest possible start for the job at that point is completion of the latest of its prerequisites. Thus, although F takes only two days, D's earliest possible start is A's finish (6). The earliest finish possible for each path is the finish of the last job on it. Normally, the early finish of the longest line's last job becomes the project time, in this case, E.

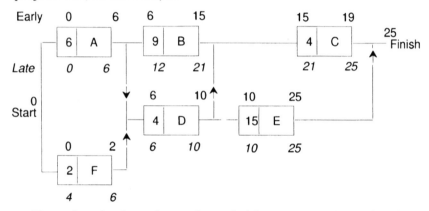

Next, do a *backward pass* from finish to start to determine *late times*, the latest time each job can be completed without extending the finish time. Put the late times under the box, as shown on the illustration above. A *critical path* is the one that takes the longest. You can tell a critical path because there is no leeway at all; that is, the late and early times are the same. In this case, it is ADE.

On segments of noncritical paths are jobs with *float time* (alias "slack" or "leeway"). There are four days of float in the F segment of the FDE path, and six days in the B-C segment of the ABC path.

Shortening Project Time

To get most efficient timing, give priority to jobs on the critical path(s) and to ones that have rigid scheduling constraints. This is like laying a rug. Cover the broad areas and trim. Then patch in the trimmed swatches to fill in the odd spaces and niches (flexible jobs with float time). In their plans of study, students fit the supervision course (offered three times a year and not a prerequisite to any other course) around key prerequisite milestones and once-a-year offerings.

If it is urgent to shorten the project, reschedule using considerations discussed earlier. One is increasing staff and other resources to shorten a long job time. World War II mobilization was an extreme application of this. Corporations were given an open-end to requisition whatever it took to get the ships and planes produced the fastest.

Another is to find critical path jobs that can be moved to a path which has float time. In the curriculum illustration used earlier, the individual therapy course has always been a prerequisite for learning group therapy, but students say the courses are so different that neither is dependent on the other. If so, we could shorten a critical path by moving group therapy to a parallel path.

A third one is a useful advanced PERT technique known as a "ladder" or a "cataract." Sometimes the whole job does not have to be completed before moving to the next one. For example, a job sequence is (1) turn out 100 right passenger doors, and (2) assemble them onto 100 cars. However, the next assembly step can get started after the first dozen are made, with subsequent doors coming on line before the first batch are exhausted. The logic is simple. The application is simple. (However, charting this makes the diagram more confusing for beginning PERTers.)

Now it is time to finish the PERT. Your final step is to allocate the float time still remaining after any adjustments to shorten the critical path. People differ on their preferences. Some may choose to do such jobs at the earliest possible time, to reduce anxiety or as a hedge against Murphy's Law. Others juggle them to balance workloads in order to minimize overtime and pressure stresses. My old roommate chose late times because he worked better under deadline pressure. (He became, appropriately, a tax accountant.) You do it your way.

A CALENDAR PERT

The project design is easier to explain to others and to follow if we convert the classical chart into a proportional horizontal calendar format. The illustration below has converted the regular PERT chart illustrated above (with float time allocated conservatively). While this illustration simply numbers from start (0) to finish (day 25), I use actual calendar dates in real life and do not schedule seven days per week.

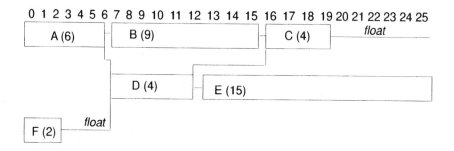

GANTT CHART

John Gantt was a pioneer scientific management expert in the early years of the century who helped the United States to mobilize for World War I. His chart is "a visual tool for work control." It is actually a matrix chart that integrates the project jobs, staff assignments, and time schedule. This can be readily adapted from the calendar chart, which already has the jobs and the time schedule. It is based on (but does not visually show) the sequencing and coordinating of jobs via paths.

There are variations in how it is presented. In one version, a horizontal calendar runs across the top, as in the calendar PERT. One which I like lists jobs (tasks) in a column down the left side of the sheet. Each job has its own line, with the job listed down the left side of the sheet, as in a traditional line item budget. The job itself is shown as a proportional box in the scheduled time spot on its line. The staff person responsible for each job is written in the box. A variation is to color code key staff and indicate responsibility by the color of the box.

A useful embellishment is to have *two* lines for each job. The top line shows the scheduled time, while the line below records the time of actual performance. This visually identifies trouble spots for early correction, as well as indicating those who are ahead of schedule and may have time available to help out in the problem areas.

TO PERT OR NOT TO PERT?

A comprehensive PERT is highly appropriate for complex macro planning. Its assets include:

- Clearly defined objectives and specific results. No wishy-washy!
- Maximum achievement: effectiveness (likelihood of success) and efficiency (best use of time and resources).
- Less hassle keeping up with everything.
- Primary prevention. It avoids problems and crises by anticipating and providing for all needs in advance (as far as humanly possible).
- Secondary prevention. With this layout, you discover and handle contingencies early, avoiding bigger problems down the road.
- Evaluation. It provides clear criteria and information to evaluate success in achieving the objective and performance by units and individuals.
- Reusability. This advantage is not normally put forth, but if you have a recurring task, such as putting out a quarterly journal or preparing courses each year, you can repeat the same basic project design with only marginal changes.
- In personal life, it can be liberating rather than restricting. By organizing tasks efficiently, you have more free time. By designing instead of playing by ear, you have more self-determination and control over how things go.

When is it least valuable? First, since it depends on accurate predictions of future circumstances, it is unreliable in situations of rapid change or instability, where there are "wicked" (non-linear) problems. It is rarely suitable for such open-ended approaches as pragmatic incrementalism, transactive planning, and learning adjustment. Finally, in a modest plan, it may be a bit of overkill. Even in all these cases, however, a little milestone PERTing never hurt anyone!

REFERENCES

Canada, Government: Regional and Economic Expansion (1982). *Project management handbook*. Ottawa.

Jackman, H. (1990). "State of the art project management methods: A survey." *Optimum* (Canada), 20, pp. 24-47.

Mulvaney, J. (1975). *Analysis bar charting*. Washington, DC: Management Planning and Control Systems.

Shelmerdine, E. (1989). "Planning for project management." *Journal of Systems Management*, 40, pp. 16-20.

IV. RELATING TO ACTORS
AND TARGETS

Are you planning for others? Are you planning *with* others? If so, what inputs do you need from them in order to set goals, determine a specific course of action, or deliver the goods? If you involve others, how will this affect your planning?

If you don't involve others, what are your reasons? It's nobody else's business: "I've made up my mind; don't confuse me with the facts"? You know more about what's best for others than they do themselves? In a hostile and competitive environment, you don't want the "enemy" to know your intents?

Participation should not be haphazard. Involvement processes are time-consuming and complicating. The Law of Parsimony says don't waste resources on unproductive participation. There are four different functions of involvement: obtaining information, enhancing the planning process, gaining support and acceptance, and enabling self-determination. Every participant should be involved for specific reasons related to one or more of the functions. Chapter 12 discusses the reasons for involvement and various bases for selection.

Overlapping with involvement is needs assessment. You can't plan without some form of it. What are goals but selected needs and wants? Chapter 13 discusses different kinds of needs as well as possible "bonus" functions of needs assessment.

Chapter 14 describes several established assessment methods. Some of them draw on traditional CRAM quantitative analysis. Others are participatory. Sections on key informants and group approaches are broadly applicable to general involvement in addition to needs assessment.

Chapter 12

Why Involve Others?

The rights and interests of every or any person are only secure from being disregarded when the person interested is himself able and habitually disposed to stand up for them.

—John Stuart Mill, *On Liberty*

The diner, not the cook, will be the best judge of the feast.

—Aristotle

WHO MAKES THE PLANNING CHOICES?

A planner can go five routes on decision making (the approaches are often mixed in large planning projects):

1. Decide for oneself.
2. Decide for others.
3. Delegate (usually subdecisions).
4. Defer to others.
5. Enable others' decisions.

Planner Decides for Self

In personal planning that takes place within accepted boundaries and does not have a significant effect on others' interests, you obviously decide for yourself. It ain't nobody's business.

Even if it does affect others, planners may still exclude them under a traditional American ideology, individualism, defined as "the pursuit of individual rather than common or collective interests." Self-interest planning considers the impact on others only to the extent that they are powerful enough to make trouble. This includes the whole range of competitive enterprise, from cornering the market on hog bellies to making the team or getting a promotion. No tears are shed for the person who lost out because you won it.

Planner Decides for Others

Plato did not believe in democracy. He experienced it in ancient Athens as irrational, capricious, unstable, and easily exploited by demagogues. He recommended a dictatorship by an expert leader. The Philosopher King is best prepared to determine the objective best interests of the people, whether or not it is what they desire. One of his disciples, Deion, actually carried this out with good results in Syracuse (until he was assassinated by his power-hungry best friend). Professional accreditation and certification bodies are philosopher kings.

When you own The Truth, is it not appropriate to decide for others? Said John Knox, founder of Presbyterianism, "A man with God is always in the majority." Classical CRAM owned Truth too: an "optimum choice" derived from technical analysis of data.

We run into problems when our Truth . . . isn't. One might ask, "best for *whom* in this real world of competing interests?" Deinstitutionalizing the mentally ill was such an expert decision. In the short run it saved millions of taxpayer dollars and benefited many patients. Still, given the lack of alternative community support services, you wonder if it was really best for those who, unable to manage entirely on their own, became a major segment of "the homeless."

Moses asked, "But who am I that I should go to Pharaoh and that I should bring the Israelites out of Egypt?" (Exodus 3:11). (Moses went ahead, and that was the first question the Hebrews asked *him*!) If we decide what is best for others, we must come to terms with the *arrogance of the planner.* We do not, indeed cannot, know all the facts and consequences. We are indelibly tainted by our own biases.

We cannot totally prevent the intrusion of our own rationalized interests. What gives us the right to play God?

Before you disqualify yourself, consider the rebuttal: Yes, but if not I, then who? Anyone else who makes the decision will have those deficiencies too. You *may* be the best available choice! If you default on making the decision, you have given your proxy to others who do choose to act. If they are more self-serving, biased and arrogant than you, does your default make you morally accountable for the consequences?

One thing is clear. The more you personally *do* make the planning choices, the more intensely you must address the considerations and dilemmas explored in earlier chapters on ethics and VIBES.

Planner Delegates Subdecisions

A compromise is to make broad decisions and then decentralize or delegate the specifics to others who are "closer to the action." From the mission and master strategy level, you may delegate the mid-range planning. Federal block grant programs do this. Each state develops its own plan within a given set of goals and standards. In a corporation, this delegation is to subsidiary program executives. The middle manager may decide specific objectives, then delegate the nitty-gritty implementation decisions and actions to a project manager.

Sometimes the delegation is horizontal rather than vertical. Subgroups within the National Association of Social Workers disagreed on the association's priorities. One group stressed social justice, another clinical enhancement, and a third members' job status and salary. Their solution was to develop three policy-planning-program paths, each with different subconstituencies, leadership, and staffing, within the boundaries set by the overall association.

Planner Defers to Others

In *subordinate planning*, a formal authority may give the planner marching orders. It is the normal position of a civil servant, a military officer, or an executive accountable to a board. This planning role places a premium on technical competence.

Informal-system de facto direction is also widespread, as in the case of an incremental planner who adapts his or her decisions to the political and/or economic market, and indeed any planner who operates with bounded rationality. It is less explicit than in corporate or military planning, but these planners too accept a superior authority: dominant values, cultures, and power interests. Saul Alinsky's oft-quoted Golden Rule is, "He who has the gold makes the rule."

Another kind of authority to which a planner may defer is *arbitration*. The rules of the game are laid out, with referees to enforce them. Decisions to resolve conflicting interpretations and applications of the rules are determined by referees such as parents, mentors, judges, or voters.

Planner Enables Others' Decisions

This route is a middle ground synthesis between deciding and deferring. It has a *procedural* value that the specific decision itself is less important than informed self-determination. This is the concept of the servant-leader: "You know that in the world, rulers lord it over their subjects, and their great men make them feel the weight of authority. But it shall not be so with you. Among you, whoever wants to be great must be your servant" (Matthew 20:25).

Among the enabling methods are:

- Empowerment of new decision makers, as in community organization, social development, and grassroots advocacy planning: enabling actors to develop *their* analytical skills, self-esteem, assertiveness, verbal communication, and social process skills.
- Facilitating the decision process through democratic task group process, conflict resolution techniques, coalition building methods, etc.
- Technical assistance, especially information and data analysis, to enable informed decisions. This ranges from simply identifying alternatives, to listing their pros and cons, to recommending a choice with reasons given.
- Organizational and managerial services.

One blend of CRAM analysis and enabling is *indicative planning*, which provieds data analysis and recommends actions but leaves decision makers free to use these inputs as they please. For instance, Wildavsky (1973) reported that "French plans have been indicative, that is, essentially voluntary. While efforts are made to reward those who cooperate, there are no sanctions for failure to comply. French plans indicate the directions wise and prudent men would take, if they were wise and prudent."

DEAL: WHOM TO INVOLVE

Planning is not haphazard. Neither is the selection of whom to involve. Everyone involved in planning decisions should be chosen for one or more specific functional reasons. The overall involvement should provide for contributions from diverse participants, covering all the bases among them.

Involvement varies at different levels of planning. Each needs different inputs from participants: sometimes focusing on desirability, other times on feasibility; sometimes emphasizing vision, other times technical knowledge. The many functions can be grouped into four clusters–Data, Enhancement, Acceptance, Liberty–the DEAL functions:

1. *Data:* information.
2. *Enhancement* of the planning process.
3. *Acceptance* and support from actors in order to succeed.
4. *Liberty* ("freedom from arbitrary or despotic control"); that is, self-determination for those affected.

Data

Planning needs lots of data. One reason for involvement is to get information that is not otherwise adequately available. It comes in three forms: raw, processed, and digested.

Raw information is direct from the sources. This may include involvement through representation, dialogue, or polling of grassroots consumers (patients, students, customers, riders) and line workers (nurses, teachers, sales reps, bus drivers). Much of this information is anecdotal fodder for insight, and a reality check on the accuracy of the processed information.

Processed information is data which has been collected, analyzed, and summarized, usually statistically. In addition to published secondary data from such sources as the census, labor statistics, and vital statistics, it may include targeted data from specific social research projects and provider agencies. If done properly, this is invaluable "hard" data, but it is restricted to that which is quantifiable and has actually been measured.

Digested information has been consumed and metabolized into theories, models, hypotheses, proposed solutions, or wisdom. Sources of this include recognized experts, key informants, community opinion leaders, and advocates. It is often the best holistic perspective on needs and possible courses of action, desirability, and feasibility, but is, of course, limited by the digester's selective knowledge and slants.

Cross-checking raw, processed, and digested information against each other should give better planning knowledge than any one or two alone. This requires multiple involvements, since the sources of each kind are usually different people.

The same diversity applies to kinds of information needed for planning. Among key types are:

- *Empirical:* substantive facts about the planning area (situation, problems, issues), including any specialized technical sub-areas.
- *Normative* indicators of the perceived needs, wants, desires, preferences, and values. This may be needed in regard to sponsors, constituents, targets, and others with a stake in the outcome.
- *Feasibility* information on existing resources, conditions of obtaining them: pragmatic constraints and limitations, laws, political factors, and obstacles. It includes intelligence about what to expect from key actors.

Enhancement

In addition to information, we involve persons who can contribute to the process of the planning itself. They should complement and enhance the package of skills the particular planner brings.

Not the least is *thinking skills*. You may want to involve persons who have particular talents for technical and mathematical analysis, integrating material into conceptual frameworks, down-to-earth common sense about applications, and/or creative thinking and vision.

If the planning involves collaboration, look for participants who have skills to facilitate *task group process*. These include *socio-emotional* and group maintenance skills, such as drawing out quiet participants, nurturing participants, defusing tension and hostility, and building cohesion.

Another set of skills contribute to *task achievement*. In addition to procedural expertise, these may include the ability to summarize a scattered discussion, suggest resolutions of conflicts, and move the group toward closure.

Acceptance and Support

The success (or failure) of most plans is influenced by an array of forces in their environments. This particularly includes actors who affect the outcomes.

Supporters legitimize and empower the plan. Formal support is needed from sponsors, boards, bosses, and constituencies. Informal sources of support may include powerful interests, the planner's reference groups (peers, a profession, a religion, a political party), and opinion leaders within the setting. Sometimes potential *dis*approvers are involved with the aim of converting or neutralizing them.

Deliverers are the ones who make it happen. They are program agencies, executives and staff, legislators, grant and contract givers, cooperating organizations, and other implementers.

Unless you are prepared to ram it down their throats, you need *acceptance* by *users*. Customers, consumers, patients, or clients may choose to accept or reject the plan's products or services. Even when targets are coerced, passive resistance can greatly diminish its effectiveness.

Passive acceptance (nonopposition) may be sufficient for potential negative forces, such as regulatory authorities, affected bystanders, and some opponents. They need only to be neutralized sufficiently not to block the plan.

Selling

One approach to support is to sell an idea *after* the decision has been made. This is euphemistically called "human engineering."

An old United Way PR man defined public relations as "doing a good job and getting credit for it." The simplest approach to selling is to have a good plan and do *rational persuasion* on its merits. While it is fashionable to pooh-pooh this as naive, it has worked for me a majority of the time, particularly on matters of relative indifference to the other's interests. It does less well with vested interests unless a persuasive enlightened self-interest case can be made.

Manipulation

Deceptive and manipulative selling is not uncommon. At its crudest, there are *outright lies* about the purpose and predicted effect, as in the successful 1981 plan to redistribute the tax burden from the wealthy to the middle and working classes, which was sold as "neutral simplification." (It was neither neutral nor a simplification.)

A more subtle approach is to *manipulate* ("to manage and control artfully or by shrewd use of influence"). A widely used manipulation is *irrational persuasion*, good ol' Madison Avenue MR (motivational research). As in the typical beer, auto, or cosmetic commercial, you manipulate the social-emotional side of your sales target by playing upon fantasy, image, ego, prejudice, and anxiety.

A relatively benign manipulation is to defuse the opposition by giving them a chance to get *catharsis* ("discharge of pent up and unacceptable emotions") on something expendable, after which you can take advantage of their emotional need to rebuild relationships. You can also benefit from developing personal friendships and commonalities with opponents. If the parties don't want to antagonize each other, mutual accommodation is more possible.

Coopting

An alternative is to draw competing interests into an open give–and–take political or market format of open negotiation and exchange. Unlike selling, the decision is still open when the process takes place.

Coopt (co-opt) comes from Latin word *cooptare,* "to choose together." It is "the process of absorbing new elements into the leadership or policy-determining structure of an organization as a means of averting threats to its stability of existence." In its true form, it is one of the cornerstones of successful planning. Selznick (1949) coined the term to describe David Lilienthal's successful community involvement in the TVA (Tennessee Valley Authority), one of the largest comprehensive planning projects ever undertaken.

Coopting usually takes place after preliminary planning but before decisions are final. It is a two–way street. The planners lay out their preliminary ideas about priorities, goals, objectives, and courses of action. The stakeholders (whoever will be affected) express their interests, feelings, cultural values, fears, etc. A dialogue goes back and forth. The aim is a collaborative consensus.

Where full agreement is not achievable, some accommodations are made and nonconcessions are respectfully explained. This creates a *"loyal opposition"* who accept process results they may not fully agree with because they believe their views had a fair hearing, turning potential opponents into allies or neutrals. (This doesn't preclude their trying to change the plan later on.)

Liberty

To secure these rights, governments are instituted among men, deriving their just power from the consent of the governed.

—Declaration of Independence

Liberty is "power or right of doing, thinking, speaking, etc. according to choice." In the 1960s, the "maximum feasible participation" movement sought *active* self-determination by the targets who were being planned for, not only through partisan advocacy planning but as players with a seat at the planner's table. In the 1960s, this explicitly included special advisory committees as well as self-selected representation on boards of directors.

This is more self-determination than our Founding Fathers wanted. Mistrusting the judgment of the small farmers and working class, their plan for the United States was a system in which the inferiors should elect their "betters" to represent them more wisely than they themselves would, subject to a passive acceptance known as "*consent*," exercised by voting for or against them when they stood for reelection. Many planners today see this as proper for dealing with the general public.

Planners disagree on whether this is also sufficient self-determination for those who will be directly affected by the plan. How much should they share in the decision making? There are no clear rules. In competitive and adversary planning, participation from outside the group may be nil. In a collegial setting it may be high. In coopting, everyone who wants to can have an honest-to-gosh effect on the plan, at least around the edges.

REPRESENTATION

Not all individual stakeholders can be directly involved. The logistics would be overwhelming. The standard solution is a republican (small "r") approach, in which the "will of the citizens is exercised by representatives chosen directly or indirectly by them."

Who is represented? A *constituency*, "a body of supporters, customers, etc.; a clientele." It may be an *organized* body: a corporation, a labor union, the American Medical Association, the Chamber of Commerce, the American Association of Retired Persons, a neighborhood association. It may be an *unorganized* aggregation: residents in the path of a proposed new expressway, single parent families, the mentally ill.

There are a number of ways in which "representatives" are selected. The method used can make a big difference in whether and how they serve various DEAL functions. Below are identified nine common methods of selection, which are grouped into four clusters.

Organizational Representatives

1. Official

The group elects or appoints the representative, who is directly accountable back to the constituency. The representative's first commitment is to his or her subgroup, with general welfare and planning goals subordinate. A key function of such representatives may be information on normative preferences, building bridges for support and acceptance, and enhancing self-determination.

2. Quasi-Official

The person is selected by the planners on the basis of formal group leadership position, such as president or executive. For example, a state mental health human resources planning committee included the heads of major mental health agencies and of mental health professional training programs. This method is good for data of all kinds, and a key approach in seeking support and acceptance. Because of their positions, quasi-official representatives may be even more constituency-oriented than elected ones. This approach lends itself well to the Banfield (1955) political planning and Lindblom 1959 partisan mutual adjustment planning approaches discussed in Chapter 8, for the representatives are professional deal makers.

Unselected Individuals

3. Grassroots

Advocacy and transactive planning emphasize self-selection by any persons within the community who are interested enough to participate. This method is high on raw data, normative preferences, and self-determination. A limitation is that there is no way of knowing whether they accurately reflect their peers. Indeed, you can be certain that they are not typical, for the average person doesn't get involved! When this is allowed for, grassroots volunteers offer something no one else can.

4. Random Polling

This approach may provide the least-biased representation attainable. Participants are not chosen by the planners nor by their own individual ambition. They are a random cross-section sample. In some ways this may be the most reliable source of raw data, preferences, and therefore indirect self-determination. On the other hand, its reliability is always diminished by unavoidable "slants" in the selection of what questions to ask and how they are asked. Perhaps more important, it is a one-way street with no opportunity for dialogue with the planners or participation in the decision-making process.

Attributed Representativeness: Members

5. Typical

The planners select a representative perceived to be similar to the average member of the constituency. Unfortunately, in most of the cases I've seen, a "typical" member is someone whom the planners feel most comfortable with, which almost surely is *atypical* of any constituency that differs significantly from them. A local church appointed an articulate youth who could "dialogue" comfortably on an adult level to represent teenagers on its board. Is that typical of fifteen-year-olds? Or was he in fact chosen because he wasn't typical?

6. Internal Key Informant

This is a constituency member identified as a someone who knows a lot about his or her group. In a health care needs assessment of Omaha's "invisible" Latino community some years ago, the project director started by asking a friend, the proprietor of a popular Mexican restaurant-bar, "Who knows the community?" A priest and two or three customers were named, and introductions made. After each interview, the director asked for further leads until the names started repeating. Their insights were used to complement processed secondary data and a survey.

7. Opinion Leader

The planner selects people who are publicly recognized as opinion leaders within the constituency, such as a neighborhood pastor, the ward representative on the city council, or a tribal elder. They are drawn in for their ability both to reflect what "their people" really want and to deliver their support and acceptance. This may or may not be an accurate assumption. For example, the elder and the pastor may be in close touch with the grassroots, while the council member may have only superficial ties to the "common folk."

Attributed Representation: Nonmembers

8. External Key Informant

The primary reason for this selection is data, including raw (anecdotal), processed (statistics), and digested (expertise). This would include such sources as a newspaper reporter, a service provider, or a professional expert in the subject area. If there is a choice of experts, choose the one who can best contribute to additional functions such as enhancement or acceptance-support functions.

9. Advocate

This is an advocate for the interests of a constituency of which he or she is not personally a member. Depending on the planning area, this may be a cardiologist, a researcher, a teacher, a social worker, an advocacy planner, a social justice lawyer, or a Junior League committee chairperson.

Intensity of Representation

In choosing participants, a significant factor may be intensity of representativeness in each category (and in each individual).

At one end of the continuum is a representative rigidly bound to the constituency's interests and preference. The representative's primary function is to negotiate the most satisfactory outcome for them. Usually, this is good for information and preference inputs, and for negotiating with power groups, but not so good for innovative thinking or central decision-making roles.

At the opposite end is the loose representative who is primarily oriented to the broader planning purposes, with a reasonably fair outcome for his or her own constituency. A person at this end may be particularly desirable for process enhancement.

Nine national voluntary organizations cosponsored grant- funded local demonstration projects for diversion of delinquents from the courts to voluntary youth agencies. Five of the projects were chaired by a "tight" quasi-official agency representative. They all did a creditable job, in which each agency got a piece of the pie and used it satisfactorily. Two projects became demonstrations of innovative interagency collaboration. The latter were chaired, respectively, by a Junior Leaguer and a Council of Jewish Women leader, for both of whom the planning goal took precedence over constituency self-interest.

Of course, there is a lot of middle ground where participants represent constituency wants and interests substantially, but with a degree of openness and flexibility toward common interests as well. This is the essence of planning under the "pluralistic-collaborative" worldview.

Multiple Representation

> No one can serve two masters.
> Either he will hate the one and love the other,
> or he will be devoted to the one and despise the other.
>
> —*Matthew 6:24*

Ah, but nearly everyone does serve two or more, and this complicates participation. For instance, on the Christian Life and Work Division Board of the National Council of Churches, one member wore five hats:

1. *Official* appointee from his denominational office.
2. *Quasi-official* as executive secretary of a network of church-related hospitals and homes.
3. *Typical*, the only professional social worker on the board.

4. *Expert key informant* as a former Federal policy official.
5. *Advocate* of the National Welfare Rights Organization (NWRO), for whom he coordinated Protestant church support.

"Know thyself," said the inscription on the ancient oracle at Delphi. You need to be self-aware of your own multiple hats, and set criteria and priorities for how you will resolve these tensions. The above member varied with each agenda item. When his constituencies coincided, no problem. When they disagreed, he usually supported their positive interests but not their "anti" positions. For instance, he supported his agencies in support of the charitable tax deduction and purchase of service, but not in their opposition to public welfare reforms advocated by NWRO.

About 300 B.C., Menander took issue with the oracle: "In many ways the saying 'know thyself' is not well said. It were more practical to say, 'know other people.'" He was right. Planners must know where the participants are "coming from." Be aware of which hat they are wearing at a given moment. Use this knowledge to advantage to maximize their contribution to planning, and to assess its value for the plan. In addition, knowing "where they are at" can be of strategic value in pursuit of building their acceptance and support of the plan.

WHAT PARTICIPANTS BRING

Representation is not the only basis for involvement, nor is participation just a matter of plugging in the right human appliances to perform the needed functions. The darn trouble with people is that they tend to act like people. To the extent necessary (and feasible), do a profile review on each key participant.

Such a profile review can pay off in three ways. First, since each participant has a functional role, you must find persons whose particular strengths coincide with a needed function.

Second, a broad profile may identify ability to perform multiple functions. For instance, an expert may also be a skilled task group facilitator and a good clarifier. A grassroots member may be a good source of raw information, a contributor to self-determination, and a source of wise insights.

Third, every participant will have deficiencies and liabilities. It is good to anticipate them. If they are destructive, you may want to find someone else instead. If you can't avoid that liability, and it is potentially troublesome, you can look for another participant with counteracting assets. A key task group had an able but dominating person who suppressed input from the other members. The administrator kept him on the task force for his many good ideas, but appointed a highly-skilled new chair who could contain him in a gentle but firm way. This opened up the group to full participation, and also converted the problem member into an asset.

Below is a partial, suggestive listing of the kinds of things people bring with them as baggage—good, bad, and indifferent. Review this and then develop your own checklist.

Biasing Factors

In additional to recognized representation of a constituency, individuals bring many biasing factors, some of which have been discussed in the chapter on VIBES. Among these are *beliefs*, *values*, and *ideologies*:

- Professed.
- De facto: as actually practiced.
- Areas of inconsistency and ambivalence.

There are many *reference points* which influence members' thinking and perspectives:

- Sociocultural background.
- Demographic identification: gender, ethnicity, generation.
- Relationship networks: family-related, workplace, community, religious, social activities.
- Role models: parents, mentors, coaches, successful public figures.
- Sources of self-esteem: peers, family, higher status groups.
- Socialization to occupational-professional norms.
- Information sources: accuracy, completeness, gaps, slants.
- Personal vested interests: career, financial, social, ego.

Power and Status Factors

Vertical factors involve inequalities of power and influence:

• Internal position, rank, authority within the organization or group.
• Outside power and leverage over other participants, such as a superior officer in relating to other servicepersons serving on a local church board.
• Outside power over the group's ability to achieve its objectives, such as certification, regulatory approval, funding.
• Attributed higher status: associated rank (the colonel's wife), traditional authority (a priest), prestige of wealth and social class.

Horizontal factors involve acceptance and belonging. They may include:

• Identification with, or difference from, other members demographically: age, gender, class, ethnicity, religion, region of origin.
• Common memberships: club, church, alumni/ae tie, professional association.
• Symbols of belonging: style of dress and grooming, language, manners.
• Credibility, based on reputation (a long-time community volunteer), credentials (a PhD), or traditional integrity status (an auditor).

Process Skills and Qualities

Examples of process assets which may contribute to the enhancement function:

• Perspective: detached objectivity, broader context insights.
• Creative vision: "I dream what never was and ask why not."
• Analytical skills: research, planning, ability to synthesize pieces into a related whole, ability to clarify choices.
• Stimulation: initiative, provocativeness, questioning, playing devil's advocate, challenging, drawing out quiet members.

- Mediation: ability to defuse tension and hostility, negotiating skills, creativeness about alternative solutions.
- Procedural expertise: parliamentarian, discussion moderator.
- Intragroup communication skills: presentation, persuasion, discussion, recording.
- Outside communication skills: reporting, public relations, selling.
- Supportiveness: empathy, nurture, encouragement, positive feedback.
- Cohesion building: creating group norms and symbols, highlighting commonalities, role modeling mutuality and collaboration.

You may want to identify negative qualities too, in order to anticipate how to minimize or offset them. You already know them all too well from past experiences.

Personal Characteristics

Personal characteristics may have a far greater effect on planning than the rational analytical model formally recognizes. This is especially applicable in participatory areas. Some of the personality factors which affect a task group's functioning:

- Ego needs and how they are met: through acceptance, appreciation, control, or achievement?
- Level and style of assertiveness: open and easy, passive, explosive.
- Level of hostility, and how it is expressed.
- Social interaction patterns: aggressive, dependent, outgoing, shy.
- Level of emotional maturity and security.
- Level of interest—or boredom.
- Sense of humor—or lack of.

KINDS OF INVOLVEMENT

In much of this chapter, there has been an implicit premise that the participation was through various kinds of task groups. "It ain't necessarily so." Much involvement is of single individuals as informants, consultants, etc. Indeed, since the groups are a bigger can of worms, the Law of Parsimony might advise us to assume individual involvement as the default setting. Use groups only when you can give a good reason (which is quite often).

Participation can be ad hoc or continuing. *Ad hoc* means "to that." Such participation is usually one time, such as a poll questionnaire, a key informant interview, a special workshop, or the October program of a continuing group. It may be extended to a follow-up or two.

Continuing advisory participation may involve a project consultant, staff, or an advisory committee. Continuing participation with authority will probably include bosses and a board or steering committee. (Ad hoc and continuing advisory methods are elaborated in Chapter 14.)

In selecting participants, take three steps in order:

1. Be clear about the intended function.
2. Decide the method(s) to be used.
3. Consider whom to involve in light of both (1) and (2).

WHO NEEDS IT?

It is clear that everyone whom you involve in your planning and decision making brings a mixed bag of rational, nonrational, and not infrequently irrational "contributions." Then there is diversity to muddy the water. Where two or three are gathered together . . . there will be four positions.

Who needs this can of worms? Not everyone. In simple personal or compartmental planning, there is no need for outside self-determination involvement. Your need for information and expertise can be met by yourself, or at most by seeking some information and counsel from an individual or two without getting into group dynamics. On the matter of acceptance and support, you may need to consider pragmatic tactical involvement. For instance, for the best plan of study, a student needs information and counsel from an open-minded, knowledgeable advisor. If the plan includes anything exceptional, the student may also need to coopt an instructor in the subject area to assure acceptance of the plan.

Even in broader plans, not everyone welcomes involvement. For elitist planners who already "know" what is best, involvement is a pain. It opens Pandora's box. It can create opposition where there was none before. It may force compromises. It raises unfulfilled expectations. It may lengthen the planning process.

Competitive planners couldn't care less about anyone else's self-determination. What they want is absence of opposition, which is best accomplished by not letting others in on their planning. The last thing they need is someone who might blow a whistle on them or telegraph their plans to competitors.

Most major planning efforts need participation. Accountability prevents us from going our own way alone. Our information is insufficient without the knowledge and experience of others closer to the issue. Our ethics require involvement of targets. Prudence dictates involvement of key actors who can make or break the plan's success. Our only choice is to do it, as well as we reasonably can. After a stormy, conflict-ridden Constitutional Convention in 1787, Ben Franklin made a compelling closing appeal for unanimous approval. It is a fitting conclusion to our discussion of involvement.

> I confess that there are several parts of this constitution which I do not at present approve . . . [but] I agree to this Constitution with all its faults . . .
>
> When you assemble a number of men to have the advantage of their joint wisdom, you inevitably assemble with those men, all their prejudices, their passions, their errors of opinion, their local interests, and their selfish views. From such an assembly can a perfect production be expected? It therefore astonishes me, Sir, to find this system approaching so near to perfection as it does.

REFERENCES

Banfield, E. (1955). "Notes on a conceptual scheme." In Meyerson, M. and Banfield, E. (Eds), *Politics, planning, and the public interest.* NY: Free Press, pp. 303-329.

Ketcham, R. (Ed.) (1986). *Anti-federalist papers and the constitutional convention debates.* New York: Mentor (New American Library), pp. 176-177.

Lindblom, C. (1959). "The science of mudlling through." *Public Administration Review,* pp. 79-88.

Selznick, P. (1949). *TVA and the grass roots: Democracy on the march.* Berkeley: University of California.

Wildavsky, A. (1973). "If planning is everything, maybe it's nothing." *Policy Sciences,* 4, pp. 127-153.

Chapter 13

Needs Assessment: Why?

Nothing is there more friendly to a man than a friend in need.

–Plautus, 200 B.C.

WHAT IT IS

Needs assessment (NA) is collection and analysis of research and other data

  . . . to determine the nature and extent of specific need,
  . . . in a defined population of a defined geographical area,
  . . . under existing (or projected) circumstances,
  . . . in comparison with a standard of satisfactoriness,
  . . . in order to guide future interventions.

In business, the parallel function is *market analysis*.

NA usually focuses on the *unmet* portion of needs, ignoring needs perceived to be fully met, on the assumption that there is no need for further intervention. Sometimes, especially in business planning, NA may also check whether a need is oversupplied. If so, it can be cut back or discontinued to free up resources for something with a higher need priority and/or a better payoff.

It is impossible to plan without some kind of needs assessment. However, its scope may vary. It can be simple and quick, yet effective. In planning a move to the suburbs, it may be no more than sitting down for a few minutes to list (1) needs (four bedrooms/two baths, good public schools, and convenient to a commuter train), and (2) nonessential wants (landscaping, gas furnace, jacuzzi, walk to school and station). We narrowed consideration to prospects which met all the needs. From among them, we select the one which best meets the additional wants.

NA for incremental planning looks at partially met needs of existing programs (a clinic, public housing, sewage disposal). Where are they not meeting the need? Waiting lists at the clinic are evidence of demand which implies that the product is good but in short supply. If the opposite is true (vacancy rates in the housing project), NA will explore whether (a) there are too many providers leading to an oversupply, or (b) that program's poor quality is deterring persons who have the unmet need. Adjustments are made to increase or decrease provision, improve the service, or market it better.

Major developments, such as a new product, overhaul of an obsolete program, or macro community ventures (urban renewal, modernizing the infrastructure), call for a more comprehensive NA/market analysis. As the magnitude grows, more factors must be taken into account, the importance of accuracy increases, and the costs of error multiply. Building a new hospital requires more NA than adding a physician to a group practice.

Needs assessment functions at three different planning stages, each needing something a little different. You can do it separately in each stage or plan one NA to serve all of the purposes.

At the global vision level, its function is to identify the gap between "what is" and "what should be." Available data, observation and experience, and a few key informants may be enough to verify a broad hole to fill.

At the strategic level, classical NA is central to designating specific areas of unmet need as Key Result Areas, and choosing midrange goals to meet them.

At the tactical level, NA is a nuts and bolts assessment to determine specific needs/wants which the program can meet and clients will use. It looks at specific actual or potential consumers, and how well (if at all) their needs are being met within the existing state of the art, programs, and resources invested.

NEGATIVE AND POSITIVE NEEDS

A need is "something required, useful or desired." An unmet need adds the modifier, ". . . which is lacking."

Negative Need: Problems to Solve

When we think of need, we usually envision it as negative: a problem. In the traditional medical model, health and well-being are the absence of disorders. The purpose of intervention is to cure the disorder, solve the problem, fill the deficit. On the other hand, "If it ain't broke, don't fix it."

Public health has three stages of intervention for a negative need:

- *Tertiary treatment:* acute care of a fully developed problem (heart bypass surgery, rehabilitation, long-term maintenance.) Tertiary planning may be a response to an earthquake, urban blight, pollution of Lake Erie, downtown traffic gridlock, a broken marriage.
- *Secondary prevention:* catching an incipient ("in the first stages of existence") problem before it becomes acute. The Maternal and Child Health program instituted "EPSDT" as its priority: Early Periodic Screening, Diagnosis, and Treatment. Secondary prevention of the heart problem might be a test for high cholesterol level followed by a plan to reduce it before it clogs an artery. A city may modernize and expand a still-functional water system which will be inadequate within a few years.
- *Primary prevention:* keeping the potential problem from ever occurring. A respiratory primary prevention plan might include nonsmoking and clean air enforcement. Eisenhower's rural Interstate Highway plan was planned as primary prevention of future congestion.

Tertiary approaches assess population at need. Primary prevention assesses population at risk. Secondary prevention looks at both populations.

Positive Need: Enhancement

A positive need is not required but *is* useful or desirable. *Enhancement* is "an active assertive process of creating conditions and/or personal attributes that promote the well-being of people." It is opportunity-oriented and developmental: making okay things better still. Holistic health stresses fitness, not just absence of disorders. We can adapt the public health model to fit positive need:

• *Tertiary:* response to existing opportunities. After World War II, businesses responded to pent-up demand for cars and appliances. A nonprofit agency responds to an RFP (Request for Proposals) in its existing area of competence.
• *Secondary:* early identification and response to an emerging change. Japan's market share in electronics is due to an early developmental response to new American technology (which American companies declined).
• *Primary:* creating an opportunity which isn't there yet. Columbia, MD was designed as a total, balanced community and built from scratch in a cornfield. Many older students are persons who have made a primary opportunity choice to develop a dramatically different second career.

WHAT KIND OF NEED?

Before doing a needs assessment, you have to decide what you mean by need in this case. Is it a broad macro condition (sanitation) or an individualized condition (medical treatment)? Is it a negative problem (unemployment) or positive opportunity (proposed new university programs)? Are you concerned with objective or subjective needs? With documented active demand or potential demand?

There are several different criteria used to determine need. They cluster into objective, subjective, and behavioral definitions. If you mix types of need (which often makes sense), take special pains to distinguish which is which and how you will deal differentially with them.

Objective Need

Objective definitions of need are "detached, impersonal, dealing with things external to the mind rather than personal feelings." They use measurable external standards applied across the board. Hunger is subjective; malnutrition is objective.

Normative means "reflecting the assumption of a standard, model or pattern." Normative need definitions are *absolute*, "free or independent of anything extraneous." It is set by some authority: government, a profession, social scientists, regulatory agencies, "experts." To be objective it must be measurable, usually by quantitative indicators. Entitlement programs, to which people have legal rights, have to be normative to prevent individual favoritism or discrimination.

The "poverty line" is a normative needs standard. So are a high school diploma, a job, a daycare staff-to-children ratio, or a gallons-per-resident guideline for the new water system.

Relative need is *comparative*. The federal matching rate for welfare and Medicaid programs varies according to the per capita income of each state. As originally developed, those at or above the U.S. median received 50 percent reimbursement. Poorer states were reimbursed at that 50 percent plus the percentage by which they fell below the national average. The rationale was that poorer states had a greater need for federal assistance.

Subjective Need

Objective needs are determined externally. Subjective needs are internal perceptions, "relating to a thing as it is known in the mind." It is a *felt* need.

Felt needs may be internalized from external norms and comparisons. If one accepts Metropolitan Life's chart, exceeding the weight range for one's height and age may create both a normative and a felt need to reduce. If you have a moderate income but socialize with affluent friends, you may have a comparative felt need for more.

Felt needs may come from a subculture norm. In one three-generation family, both grandparents had graduate professional degrees. All five of their children had a felt need for post-college education. So did most of their grandchildren. In another family with comparable native ability, no one in the same three generations felt a need for college at all.

Felt needs may be independent of, or even contrary to, externals. If you feel hunger or pain or loneliness, you do not need outside authorities or comparisons to give you a felt need. Felt needs are usually rational, but they can be irrational too. Anorexia is a disorder in which even emaciated individuals have a felt need to reduce.

A positive felt need is a *want*, "a wish or desire for something." Ever after my first visit to Cape Cod, I had a want for a home at the beach.

When needs are assessed, *utility* is the measure of felt needs. It is defined as "the capacity of an object for satisfying a human want." While economics has narrowed this to things that money can buy, the generic term covers anything that increases happiness and well-being.

Expressed Need: Demand

Expressed means "made known, clearly indicated." It is a felt need plus some kind of reaching out to get it. This is measurable in such ways as being a current consumer/client, seeking it (making inquiries, wait listed), responding to outreach (advertisements, recruitment), or militantly insisting that a need be met.

In the economic (commercial) market, this is called *demand*, "desire for a commodity together with the ability to pay for it." In the social market of public and nonprofit services, it is being willing and able to use it . . . and *somebody* is willing and able to pay for it (through direct fees, third-party payments, tax subsidies, or charity).

There is also *potential* demand. This is an objectively assessed need for which active expressed need could be created if:

- People become aware of their needs/wants through such means as diagnosis, referral, education, consciousness raising, or advertising.
- People learn that something can be done about it.

- People find out that the service exists or may be developed soon.
- People discover that the service is accessible in terms of location, cost, office hours, transportation, language, and culture.

WHAT POPULATION?

Set the geographic boundaries for your assessment (a census tract, the standard metropolitan area, a five-county region, the nation). Set demographic boundaries relevant to the specific need, such as age (infants, senior citizens, teens), gender, income, ethnicity, family status, educational level.

Beyond this, a key distinction in needs assessment is whether you are looking at the population at *need* or the population at *risk.*

Population at Need

A population at need is people who currently have the condition in a tertiary or secondary stage.

Some of those at need can be identified by direct data because they are already being served by hospitals, social agencies, physicians, unemployment insurance, Social Security, special education, or the criminal justice system.

Inevitably, this will undercount the real population at need because not everyone is identified by the system. For instance, unemployment statistics count only active job-seekers. "Discouraged workers" who want jobs but have given up looking are missed. Therefore, this useful approach must be supplemented by methods to estimate the unreported need.

One is a random sample survey, which discovers the percentage of persons with the condition who are not receiving service. Based on this sample, you can statistically estimate the probable number of unidentified cases in the total population. Search the literature. Often you will find that someone else has already done a survey that is close enough to be useful for your purposes, saving you the time and expense. This is the case, for instance, regarding discouraged workers.

Another way is to take national statistics and project them to your population group. An Urban League study on "The State of Black Omaha" (Burch, 1981) discovered that local rates (life expectancy, infant mortality, tuberculosis, income, education, etc.) were consistently about average for African Americans nationally. Where local data was not available, it therefore felt reasonably confident to project the national average. On the other hand, incidence of AIDS in Omaha deviates widely from national averages, which are therefore of limited use in assessing local needs. Another factor to consider in using national statistics is how complete and accurate their sources are. Some are precise, others may be a compilation of local guesstimates.

Attributed need is sometimes a shortcut. Find easily measurable characteristics which correlate with the need. If most of the members of a categorical group have the same condition, isn't it easier and cheaper to blanket in the whole group instead of checking out each one's need? Headstart attributed need to all preschool children in its low income catchment neighborhoods. This freed up more funds for providing the service–and eliminated the stigma of being diagnosed individually as needy.

The limitation on attributed need lies in its accuracy. Headstart's attributed need is probably 90 to 95 percent accurate. Reduced bus fares for the elderly were 75 percent accurate (close enough?) when initiated, based on pre-social security poverty rates for that age group. Today, while there are still many needy elderly, the poverty rate is about one-sixth of what it was. A retired colleague whose income is twice the national average bragged to me about going from San Francisco to Berkeley for a dime. Meanwhile, single-parent households, with three times the poverty rate of the elderly, are excluded. This may be good politics, but it is not good needs assessment.

Population at Risk

For tertiary services, population at need is the way to go. If your aim is primary or secondary prevention, you want to know the population at risk (or the population with positive potential) so that you can intervene more effectively at an earlier point.

There are too many variables to pinpoint a population at risk precisely. However, you can predict a population which has the greatest probability of developing the condition eventually if you know causal factors, such as:

- *Behavior:* alcohol increases cirrhosis; sunbathing increases skin cancer.
- *Life experience:* abused children are at higher risk of becoming abusers.
- *Environment:* When I lived in New York City, a standard greeting was "How is your sinus?"
- *Genetic predisposition:* alcohol problems, schizophrenia, and breast cancer rates are higher where there is a family history of the condition.
- *Demographics:* poor people have more multiple health problems and less life expectancy.

You can also project risk from characteristics which are not causative but which covary with the need you are assessing. Nonmalignant skin blemishes may be only a cosmetic nuisance, but their presence indicates the same kind of exposure that causes skin cancer.

If you can identify the population at need with some reliability, you can plan primary and secondary prevention steps to help them avoid the conditions for which they are at risk.

IMPORTANCE OF THE NEED

Both quantity and quality enter into determining the importance of a need. There is no absolute formula that you can plug in and get the answer. As a planner, you have to weigh the different aspects in making your judgment.

Number of Cases

How many have the need (or are at risk)? This is counted two ways. Depending on the planning purpose for the NA, you may use one or the other, or both:

- *Incidence* is raw numbers. This is especially important for estimating how many persons would use a new or expanded service.
- *Rate* is the frequency of the problem, the percentage of the
  population who have it. This is especially important in making
  priority choices among competing needs.

Seriousness

The importance of a need depends on how seriously it affects the
person who has it, or the society at large.

One way to define it is *intensity* of the condition. Pimples and
pregnancy are two common teenage problems today. Although pimples have a much higher incidence, we assess pregnancy as the
priority. It's like the pig invited by a chicken to be a partner in a
ham-and-eggs breakfast business. The pig declined, saying, "For
you, it's all in a day's work, but for me it's total commitment."

Another criterion is *consequences of nonintervention*, what happens if nothing is done about it. There are several dimensions of
this:

- *The ultimate result.* Untreated, will the person at need fully re-
  cover eventually (a cold), continue impaired (arthritis), or die
  (cancer)?
- *Immediacy.* How urgent is it? What are the consequences of
  delay? A brittle diabetic without insulin may be dead in a few
  days, while a person in need of a knee replacement can survive
  a two-year waiting period, albeit with much pain and disability. A contaminated water system is an immediate threat, while
  inadequate supply may be tolerable for several years, with inconvenience and rationing, while developing new sources.
  (Faced with the latter a few years ago, a Florida Keys motto
  was, "In this land of sun and fun/We don't flush for Number
  One.")
- *Ripple effects.* What are the side effects on others? Does a clin-
  ically depressed young mother of five represent a greater need
  than a retired widower with the same condition? Is violent
  crime a higher priority than white-collar theft?

UNMET NEED

The bottom line of needs assessment is *unmet* need. For service programs, this is simple arithmetic: the total incidence minus the number currently being served adequately. This is our familiar *gap* from the BASIC model.

Quantitative Gap

The quantitative gap is the number of cases not provided for. This number includes unmet *recognized* need. There is simply not enough provision. Key documentation of this need includes waiting lists, clients turned away, and overcrowding.

NA also seeks to discover hitherto *unrecognized* need. One reason for unrecognized need is faulty diagnosis. In a deep recession a few years ago, with 20,000,000 Americans out of work, President Reagan held up the want ads section of the *Washington Post* and declared authoritatively that everyone who "really" wants to work can find a job. Based on this diagnosis, he recognized no unmet employment need, and therefore did nothing about it.

A widespread NA problem is *invisibility*. A colleague, doing a needs assessment in a rural region, asked the director of the largest human service agency about needs and services in the Native American community. The director replied, "Oh, we don't have one." "Yes you do. I've been there often." "Show me." My colleague did. The director, with a rueful smile, then pointed to a nearby grove of trees on the edge of the neighborhood and admitted, "I live on the other side of those woods, only half a mile away, and I never knew they were here!"

When the public assistance program was passed in 1935, it recognized four categories of poor people: widows and children, the aged, the blind (later adding "the permanently and totally disabled"), and temporarily unemployed men. The invisibles were men and women, often in their fifties, with marginal education and skills, without dependent children, and typically with borderline disabilities which affected their employability as unskilled workers. They were too old for employment programs and ADC (Aid to Dependent Children), but not quite old enough or disabled enough for Social Security. Legally, they simply did not exist. They are still largely invisible today. (European social insurances make special provision for them.)

An NA challenge is to discover the true extent of the need, including those overlooked due to ignorance, ideology, or indifference–or all of the above.

Qualitative Gap

A different kind of unmet need is *inadequate* provision. The need is recognized and services are being rendered, but they aren't getting the job done. This has sometimes been a problem, for example, in the nursing home industry. What is good enough to count as meeting the need?

To assess qualitative need, you have to define an explicit standard of "adequacy." As discussed in the ethics chapter, definitions vary on a continuum between "barely passable" and "fully satisfactory." There may be a discrepancy between official standards and de facto practice. My board of regents proclaims "excellence in education" as its standard but budgets instruction at "the gentleman's C" level: good enough to pass accreditation reviews respectably. Good assessment must settle on a consistent, honestly applied standard which will genuinely guide the planning. If not, don't waste your time going through the motions.

When assessing the causes of a qualitative gap, the first question is, what is the state of the art? In the 1950s, the Philadelphia Health and Welfare Council pioneered an evaluation of social agencies based on priority of need and effectiveness in meeting it. The alcoholism clinic came out number one in need and dead last in success rate. Apparently this was the "state of the art" for clinical programs at that time.

Given this assessment, you have two good choices, to forget the whole thing and reprogram resources to other needs, or to refocus your planning on research and experimental programs.

Some Community Mental Health Centers in my area take the first route. They turn away two of the most pressing mental health problems, "borderline personality" and "sociopath" because those disorders do not respond well to the kinds of therapy they offer. This frees up their limited resources for what they can do successfully.

The National Institutes of Health have historically represented the second route, responding to the same problem with funded research and experimentation. Perhaps each is making the appropriate choice for its respective situation.

Planners often do neither. In Philadelphia, with an expedient eye on public relations and fund raising, the Council refrained from expanding the alcohol program but continued to support the popular but ineffective program. At least the Council knew what it was doing and why. Too often, faulty assessments respond to unmet need by expanding existing inadequate programs. This is called by critics "throwing good money after bad" or "throwing money down a rat hole."

If the general state of the art is okay, but the qualitative gap exists anyway, the next question is whether there is something wrong with the program. Maybe it's a lousy agency. This too offers two choices. The obvious choice is to shape up the agency. Unfortunately, this is easier said than done. Entrenched staff and administrators are hard to move.

The second choice is to develop a better one to take its place. One of my students, a physical therapist, documented a need in the community for good paraplegic rehabilitation. The problem was that a poor program existed, and there were not enough cases to support two. When the existing program stonewalled, she recommended that her own hospital develop a competing quality program. It was feasible and potentially profitable. However, as is often true in such cases, they made a third choice, the traditional professional stance that in the absence of flagrant abuse, tolerating a qualitative unmet need is preferable to criticism of, or *overt* competition with, peers.

Accessibility

Sometimes, even though services to meet a need exist "on paper," the need may still be unmet because it is not *accessible*. The British National Health Service covers nonemergency surgery, but you have to sign up for it in advance. The delay can literally last a lifetime for some older patients. In other cases, a service may be available, but in a time, place, and form which you cannot use.

Some of the factors which affect the accessibility of services and benefits are listed below. The first two have been discussed.

- *Quantity.* Is there enough to go around, or will some come away empty?
- *Quality.* Are the standards such that you actually get what was promised?
- *Location.* Can clients get to it with the transportation available to them and in their physical conditions?
- *Schedule.* Can ordinary people use it without risking loss of their jobs?
- *Information.* Do people understand what is available and how to apply?
- *Affordability.* Can all "eligible" people meet the costs of getting a service, including fees, transportation, baby-sitting, lost wages, etc.? If not, can such barriers be worked out on an individualized basis?
- *Usability.* Is help offered in the client's language? Is the food kosher? Are there ramps and elevators for disabled users?
- *Acceptability.* Is it provided without stigma in a respectful, supportive manner compatible with the client's culture?

Gray Areas

It would be more comfortable if NA could give us clear-cut, unequivocal yes/no answers on need. Sometimes that is possible. A child must have schooling. There are two choices: go to school or have an approved home teaching arrangement. If neither, the need is unmet.

More often, between ideal well-being and critical deprivation lies a continuum. How good does it have to be to be considered "met"? How bad does it have to be to warrant intervention—in poverty, in socioemotional problems, in educational development?

Effectiveness of provision is a gray area. How much is enough? Does it work? At a bare subsistence level of income, education, or mental hospital care, is the need being met? Most of us say no. Does it have to be optimum (whatever that is)? Most of us wistfully say, "I guess not." Between these extremes, should it provide some enrichment and quality beyond the bare minimum? We all say yes, but argue about where to draw the line.

A related gray area exists where the quality is satisfactory but *inefficient.* This is especially important when there is an unmet need, because more people could be served if it did a better job. In a broader perspective, even if there is no unmet need in *this* area, inefficiency still diverts resources that could meet other needs.

Obviously, such NA findings point to overhauling or replacing that program. Which? Do you rebuild the engine or buy a new car? At what point is the inefficiency bad enough to warrant the latter? A good question!

Finally–and this is a perennial dilemma in the public sector– what are we prepared to trade off between quality and quantity? Higher education used to be a want, not a requirement. There was more emphasis on quality than quantity. Today, college education is considered a vocational need which should be available to most high school graduates and relatively affordable even to low-income persons. My underfunded urban university struggles with a chronic quality-for-quantity tradeoff dilemma at the freshman and sopho- more levels. Dialogue in class, independent thinking, and original papers may give way to large lecture sections and computer-graded multiple choice tests. Is it a sound tradeoff? In needs assessment, "that's where the rubber meets the road!"

MULTIPURPOSE NEEDS ASSESSMENT

The official purpose of needs assessment is to assess needs. However, there are other functions it can perform–and if it can, it should (within reason). Your information-gathering methods can be designed to advance other planning elements as well, such as coopt- ing support and acceptance, and gathering baseline data for evalua- tion, marketing, and social action.

Program Decisions

NA identifies the nature and extent of existing and projected needs: what, who, where. It should include information on caus- ative factors behind the symptoms, a critical factor for planning interventions.

You use it in strategic planning steps: identifying the desirable situation (your standard of need), the current situation, the unmet needs gap, causes, key result areas, and needs-based goals.

In combination with practical cost and feasibility analyses, it contributes toward an informed synthesis of what is desirable with what is ultimately possible at the concrete level. Why not blend some of the feasibility aspect into the NA itself by adding a "resources survey" piece?

Marketing

By locating the felt needs, wants, and demand, a good needs assessment should contribute to marketing your future product. Who would or might use your product if it were known and accessible? Whose felt needs can be activated to demand? What are key referral sources? Whom do they refer now, for what, to whom? What would attract referrals from them to your new/enhanced program? Who could/would pay for your service if offered (the consumer, a third party, a public or charitable subsidy)?

Don't just collect data. Keep an extra journal in which you note names and information about people for possible later follow-up in such areas as funding and support, recruitment and referral, interagency collaboration, or expert assistance.

It is appropriate to plow for needs in previously untilled soil (unrecognized needs). In addition to benefiting the "invisible" group, you may open a virgin lode of potential demand for which you have the inside track. A word of caution: untilled fields are often populated by people with limited ability to pay. In such cases, the NA should be paired with a serious resource assessment.

Acceptance and Support

Agencies do formal NA even when they don't really feel the need of one. Why? An old rhyme goes:

I eat my peas with honey;
I've done it all my life.
I don't like peas with honey,
But it keeps them on the knife.

Virtually every project grant made by government or charity requires a formal Needs Assessment report and documentation. My experience in federal grant programs was that although some applicants did not need one, we had to make it mandatory in order to keep from being inundated with half-baked proposals from the rest.

So . . . if you want the peas, pour the honey, whether you need it or not. You want a grant? Use your NA to justify it. You are planning a fundraising campaign? A well-documented needs-assessment rationale will soften the ground, particularly with tough-minded large donors who may see human services as dominated by "bleeding hearts." A good NA presents a program as "softhearted and hardheaded." Well, if you must do it, you might as well get full value out of it by seriously using its findings to cross-check what you already thought you knew.

To serve these dual needs, make sure that your NA information includes good "selling" data that you might not have bothered with for pure assessment. Also consider writing it up twice, first as an unvarnished assessment for planning purposes, and afterward in a promotional, marketing format.

There is another key acceptance and support function that can be blended honestly into your NA. Inevitably, many key informants are *also* key potential actors who can help or hinder your plan. Drawing them in up-front creates positive relationships, reduces hostility and mistrust, and gives them an opportunity to "own" a small piece of your plan as their own (assuming their input influences your decisions). You can lay the groundwork for future collaborations and referrals. Your information may also give you good predictions on what to expect from them, good and bad, down the road, which you will use in developing strategies and tactics.

If this is desirable for key informants, it is also desirable to add other key actors on the list for acceptance-support reasons, whether you need their information or not. This modest manipulation is ethical if you play the game honestly: whatever your reason for including them, treat them and their information exactly as you do all other informants.

Quite apart from special support efforts, the very fact of doing a needs assessment pays promotional and public relations dividends. The process makes people aware that the agency exists. "Say anything about me you want. Just spell my name right." It presents the agency as a caring, competent, aware, responsive organization. This alone should increase demand and soften the ground for possible financial support.

Evaluation

Plan your evaluation before you design the needs assessment. In addition to being a good mechanism to help you define your interests, it enables you to incorporate the baseline "before" data into the NA.

Improving Other Agencies

In the BASIC model, a selection criterion is horizontal compatibility with other agenda of the organization or planners. One agendum of public and nonprofit planners may be to educate other existing providers to improve *their* services. By drawing them in, and sharing your findings, you may help them to discover their own quality gaps and overlooked unmet needs. (This may not apply to frankly competitive enterprise.)

A group of human service middle managers in western Nebraska were frustrated that their community was not providing health care to its Mexican-American subgroup. While in fact there were major accessibility barriers, the "established" agencies comfortably assured that there was no unmet need because they were "available." The volunteers did a needs assessment (as a planning class project) that documented the unmet need. The agencies still refused to address it, so the group organized a part-time clinic under the auspices of Latino leaders at Our Lady of Guadalupe Church, with volunteer doctors and nurses. The demand was absolutely overwhelming.

With their reputations impaired and fearing loss of revenues, the old agencies initiated special outreach programs and Spanish-speaking services in competition with the new clinic. Dropping its own clinic, the project shifted to outreach services and patient advocacy with the established agencies. The ultimate result of the needs assessment was not program development by the planners but *social action* which changed community practices.

Compatible Functions

There is no need for the different uses of NA conflict. Indeed, they are complementary functions:

- Identifying needs and determining future program directions.
- Creating new felt needs and demand.
- Selling the program to potential funders, sources of referral, and users.
- Evaluation design.
- Social change through consciousness raising, sharing information, community organization, and/or putting other agencies on the spot.

REFERENCE

Burch, H. and Burch, G. (Eds.). *The state of Black Omaha.* Omaha, NE: Urban League of Omaha.

Chapter 14

Needs Assessment: Methods

How do I need thee? Let me count the ways.

—With apologies to Elizabeth Barrett Browning

Needs assessment as discussed in this chapter originated in human service planning. Its business counterpart is market analysis. It uses three mutually compatible approaches to needs assessment: available secondary data, key informants, and survey.

AVAILABLE SECONDARY DATA

Social Indicators

> The social indicators approach to needs assessment is based primarily on inferences of need drawn from descriptive statistics found in public records and reports. . . . It is possible to make useful estimates of the needs and social well-being of those in the community by analyzing statistics on factors found to be highly correlated with persons in need. (Warheit et al., 1977, p. 30)

Before going out "live," start in the library. Do not reinvent the wheel. Get information the old-fashioned way: from someone else. In the exploratory stage of a needs assessment, look up basic *social indicators*. (Warning: It is easy to get lost in such a maze of information. To avoid overkill, be clear what you are looking for and pick the right *key words*.)

You will want:

- General information about the target area and/or target population.
- Direct indicators of the incidence of the condition (out of wedlock births, diagnosed cases, sewer overflows).
- Indirect indicators that correlate with the condition (heavy drinking with cirrhosis, low education with low income).

If you are poking around unsure of what you want, a good pump primer is to scan the Federal Government's annual one-volume *Statistical Abstracts of the USA*, which contains summary tables on an incredibly wide range of topics. This in turn may lead you to *its* sources, such as the Census, the Bureau of Labor Statistics, the Government Accounting Office, criminal justice, vital statistics, and state program agency data.

Perhaps you can find someone who has already pulled together a piece of your data, such as the local United Way, the state Commission on Mexican-Americans, or a local university's social research center. In addition to having information to share, they may even gather more for you, or help you to do so.

Legitimate advocacy groups in your area of interest can be a primary source. Caution: consider the source. The responsible ones, such as the Children's Defense Fund or the Study Group on Social Security, distinguish between meticulously objective reporting of data and their value-based recommendations. Extremist groups and phony advocacy groups which are fronts for vested interests often suppress unfavorable findings, twist data in misleading ways, and even fabricate outright falsehoods. *Consumer Reports* (Consumer's Union, 1994) warns, "Industry funding compromises any claim to scientific independence."

Other sources are periodicals that offer both primary and secondhand reported data. These include law, professional, scientific, and social commentary journals, as well as newspapers and popular news magazines.

Advantages of social indicators are that they can provide extensive data readily at low cost. Because they have already been expertly processed, the user need not have extensive research-technical training.

There are limitations. Indirect indicators should not be mistaken for the actual need. There is always an imperfect correlation at best.

- Where errors about inferred causes have been made, the indicators based on them will necessarily be off base.
- Broad general background data may be excellent for strategic perspective, but by itself gives only minimal guidance on causes, possible interventions, specific courses of action, or the specific individuals who have the need.
- "Canned" data is usually kept by census tracts and/or political boundaries, which rarely coincide precisely with your geographic area of interest. To use the data, you must dilute it by including off-target populations within the census tract and dropping small pieces of the target area which overflow into largely outside tracts.

The limitations of social indicators can be offset by information gathered from other methods, cross-checking multiple sources, and maintaining a healthy skepticism (stopping short of cynicism). Where sources support each other you can have more confidence. When they conflict, investigate the reliability of the conflicting sources, get more information, and/or find an explanation that resolves the apparent conflicts.

Social indicators information is most useful for global and strategic level scans. It provides a stronger knowledge base from which to select informants and ask better questions in the rest of the needs assessment.

Epidemiology

Epidemiological studies by bodies such as Centers for Disease Control offer national information on the demographic distribution of a condition, apparent causes, and possible interventions. Often the data is broken down by states or regions, from which you can estimate incidence or rate within your planning boundaries.

Information in a RUT

Another set of useful available data comes from agencies currently serving the need. It is known as *Rates Under Treatment* (RUT), which is part of a good service agency's Management Information System (MIS). "The underlying assumption is that the needs of the community can be established from a sample of persons who have received care or treatment" (Warheit et al., 1977, p. 26).

Your first RUT source is your own organization. It should give you a profile of existing consumers: their characteristics, their presenting problems, the treatment, and the outcome. The Law of Parsimony applies to this data. On the one hand, keep all information necessary for accountability and program planning. Undercollection of essential data prevents rational evaluation and planning. On the other hand, keep it simple and brief. Overcollection can be incredibly wasteful of line worker and clerical staff time.

You may want to augment RUT statistics with a few insightful anecdotal human interest cases. Needless to say, RUT–and anecdotes–must be processed in such a way as to protect client confidentiality.

Another key source of RUT is the other providers, so that you can know the full extent of the identified need and how much of it is met within the whole community. Sometimes agencies get defensive and refuse to share information. Remind them that service statistics and budgets of public and charitable organizations are legally open to the public which supports them. If an agency refuses, you may challenge it with media exposure and/or court injunctions. (Commercial services have certain protections from disclosures which might be used to advantage by a competitor.)

Umbrella organizations and regulatory bodies that pull together service information from their affiliates may offer a one-stop RUT shortcut. A local United Way has standardized, comparable data on every agency it funds. State education, health, mental health, rehabilitation, social welfare, and justice system agencies collect annual service data from related programs.

RUT gives good information on *demand*, met and unmet, indicated by the number and outcomes of applicants. It provides "hard information" on the demographic and diagnostic characteristics of persons known to be in need. These can provide clues about what to look for to identify (1) undiscovered persons in need, and (2) populations at risk. Drop-out rates before the need is fully met are indicators of possible qualitative gaps.

In addition to gaining information, the process of collecting it is an excuse to sensitize other agencies to the unmet needs and to coopt them into a collaborative rather than competitive relationship.

RUT may be limited in the extent to which one can project from the treated group to the rest of the populations at need and risk. Half of poor elderly persons eligible for Supplemental Security Income welfare payments do not apply. A big reason seems to be pride. Many old people would rather die than "go on relief." If this is true, RUT information on the recipient half is of little value in addressing the unserved half.

RUT is good for what it is good for: a convenient, cheap way to get primary knowledge about recognized needs, persons who have them, and the adequacy of existing services.

KEY INFORMANTS

Why?

In Chapter 12 we discussed DEAL, the four functions of involvement: Data, Enhancement of the process, Acceptance and support, and Liberty/self-determination. The obvious purpose for involving key informants, as discussed here, is the Data function.

Key informants can give you a quick scan with surprising accuracy. Some years ago, parallel teams from social planning classes at Brandeis and MIT studied ten nearby communities. The Tech teams did a comprehensive review of all available data. The Brandeis teams used only the key informant method. When the two classes compared notes, the parallel teams for each town presented amazingly similar conclusions and recommendations!

Different kinds of informants serve different purposes. Target group members and line agency workers are good sources about felt need. Advocates often have contributions to make on comparative need. Agency administrators and "expert" informants are usually best on normative needs. These can be cross-checked with each other as well as surveys and secondary data. All key informants are also sources of *feasibility* information: potential support, opposition, obstacles.

In addition, as noted in Chapter 13, the selection of and approach to key informants should concurrently serve other functions. Enhancing support and acceptance should always be a conscious second function. To the extent that the planner respects their inputs, grassroots informants contribute a measure of self-determination.

Who?

Who should be an informant? That depends on what you are looking for. Among the most commonly used sources are:

- *Experts* on the needs areas, including those in university, research, and advocacy settings.
- *Providers*, such as physicians, teachers and guidance counselors, caseworkers, police, and emergency room nurses, as well as their supervisors and program directors.
- *General community leaders*, such as businesspersons, union heads, politicians, long-time volunteers, and clergy.
- *Indigenous leaders*, such as civil rights activists, PTA officers, and ward heelers.
- *Other informed persons*, such as newspaper editors or reporters. This catchall is the place to seek diversity to counterbalance the slants of other selected informants and to fill information gaps.
- *Other influential actors* whom you need to coopt for acceptance and support.

How do you identify them? One method is *outside-in*, inviting people already known to the planners because of their positions, reputations, and activities. A second is *inside-out*, in which you start with any member of a constituency and keep asking each informant you interview who else to talk to.

Before inviting any key informant, you need to determine (1) what kinds of information you want for what purposes, and (2) other functions you want to use it for. Select only persons who fit one or both of these purposes.

GROUP APPROACHES

A group is a collection of people which has the following characteristics:

- Common focus: shared purposes and activities.
- Direct personal interaction with each other.
- Moderate to substantial social-emotional relationships.
- Structure and norms about roles, procedures, behavior, and relationships, usually both explicit and evolving from the culture of the group.

Existing Groups

A key distinction is between preexisting groups, and ad hoc groups formed for this single (information) purpose.

An example of an existing group was the monthly National Association of Social Workers chapter meeting, which I visited as part of a needs assessment for the School of Social Work. There is good news and there is bad news about using *existing* groups. The bad news is it is more difficult to get what you want from the group. You come in cold as an outsider to a close-knit body with an established group culture. They, not you, are running the meeting on their terms. They often allow too little time for discussion in depth. You have no choice of participants, so you will miss some of the best potential informants and get some persons who subvert the process with digressions, hostility, or ego-emotional problems. These limitations are no big deal, provided the deficiencies are met through other sources, such as individual interviews and planner-selected ad hoc groups.

On the plus side, it is efficient and convenient. In the above case, the chapter offered ready-made access to some of the most knowledgeable and concerned professionals in the region, whose guidance and active support were essential.

Prepare carefully for existing groups, including a concise presentation that introduces them to the situation, concerns, and general directions, and gives them a framework of what information you are looking for. Your purpose is to receive their input in an open-ended way. You can probe their comments for clarity or elaboration but it is not a place to argue, promise, or propose.

A record should be kept of the information received. It is difficult to take good notes while remaining fully engaged in a sensitive group process. It can be done if you have a retentive memory that can reconstruct a whole input from a single, jotted key word.

A common practice is to tape the meeting. A verbatim recording is fine as a backup, but wasteful to transcribe and plow through. The ideal is a skilled note taker to record and organize the important kernels of wheat while letting the chaff blow away. Ideally, the recorder should also make marginal notes on nuances such as body language, voice timbre, and other indicators of whether and how one might work with the group or individual members in the future. (In task group process, these are normal "staffing" functions.)

Ad Hoc Groups

An *ad hoc* group is a one-shot affair (or at most a few meetings with a beginning and an end). This is often used as an alternative to individual interviews on the expectation that the interaction of the participants will stimulate each other more than sitting and thinking alone (often but not always the case).

In contrast to existing groups, an ad hoc group can be tailored to precise needs in subject matter, participants, and process. You can invite only the most desirable informants relative to the subject. It can address the whole plan or only a specialized area within it.

The NASW chapter was fine for broad interests, but since most of the members were direct service practitioners, it was not a fruitful setting in which to deal with the macro training subtopic (social policy, planning, administration, and organizing). It was supplemented with a specially focused ad hoc conference of leading macro practitioners on the training needed for their area.

You can have as many ad hoc groups as you choose. The example above was a topical breakdown. Another kind of breakdown may be according to different peer groups: one meeting for community leaders, another for agency heads, a third for line workers, a fourth for the client group, and a fifth for community grassroots people. You can also simply break the larger body randomly into parallel small groups to enhance participation, without reference to topics, or pair groups.

The primary function of most ad hoc informant groups is to give direct information. A complement to this can be the *feedback group*. After collecting information from individuals, separately or in a group, mail a summary of the findings (from all assessment sources) to selected informants, and invite them to a session in which they comment (and perhaps argue with each other) about the information and inferences, the program and planning implications, and how it affects their interests. In addition to insight on needs, feedback groups can provide feasibility and tactical information on probable responses from consumers, funders, and other actors.

A feedback session can be done toward the end, after your penultimate ("next to last") draft conclusions are written, or at an earlier stage before your thinking has fully jelled. If you use them at several stages, you have crossed a fine line upgrading the involvement from "informant group" to "advisory committee." Feedback groups are effective with articulate experts and leaders. They also do well with grassroots people if the planner is self-aware, has transactive skills, and doesn't try to con them.

A similar feedback process but without meetings is called the *Delphi* technique (Dalky, 1967). The multistage input and feedback dialogue is carried out through successive rounds of questionnaires, each built on and accompanied by a summary of the previous one.

Group Size

"Seminar size" is a good standard for informant groups. Both are designed for high participation and cross-pollination of ideas. The group should be large enough to provide some diversity and stimulation (say four or more), yet small enough for every member to participate fully. Beyond about a dozen, the "crowding" of discussion time begins to defeat its purpose.

What if you are stuck for various practical or political reasons with a too-large informant group? One approach is to break into interest groups. A large advisory group to our state mental health authority on future needs and priorities was divided into separate discussion groups, set up for the concerns of the several professions, paraprofessionals, and patients, with a staff person to record each subgroup. In the closing plenary session, comments on each subgroup's recommendations were invited and recorded, but no attempt was made to reach a consensus. In effect, we had several separate ad hoc groups under one roof.

A different effect can be achieved by a nonspecialized breakdown into smaller cross-section "buzz groups." This is useful with grass-roots informants and when seeking interdisciplinary dialogue. In both cases, members are likely to open up more in a small group than in the large one. A buzz group breakdown is often followed by active plenary group interaction aimed at achieving a group consensus.

What if you decide on an oversized group anyway? Michel's *iron law of oligarchy* will cut it down the hard way. It states that regardless of the size of a body, whether 15, 50, or 5,000, an inner core of six to fifteen will dominate, with everyone else on the periphery.

Group Communication Styles

Among the several common communication methods within groups, are "star," "center pivot" and "feed the kitty."

As children we drew stars with a continuous line connecting each point with the others. *Star* communication is direct back-and-forth interaction of all members with each other. This is good for creative, innovative, and problem-solving purposes, as well as working toward consensus through dialogue. On the other hand, it is more time consuming and digressive, and it requires more group process skills and sensitivity to run than other styles. Under a weak or laissez faire leader, it is vulnerable to domination by the most verbal and assertive members at the expense of deliberate thinkers and quiet ones.

Center pivot irrigation makes those circular fields (as opposed to rectangles) that you see when you fly over the plains. It has a central water source, which connects directly with every point on the perimeter through a movable pipe. A center pivot group is a leader-controlled method, such as parliamentary procedure. Each member must be recognized by the pivot (chair) and officially speaks only to this person. This is an effective style for keeping focused on an agenda, minimizing digressions, and reaching closure. It gives the leader formal power to moderate aggressive members and draw out the quiet ones—at the expense of spontaneity, creativity, and direct back-and-forth dialogue among group members. In the hands of an unskilled or undisciplined group leader, it is susceptible to overcontrol.

Feed the kitty is like anteing up in a poker game. Each person in turn lays his or her chip of input on the table for all to see, before any response is permitted. This guarantees that every member is heard. Its chief limitations are fragmentation and lack of opportunity to enhance or build ideas.

A mix may be better than any one alone. You might start with a round of feed the kitty in which everyone, bold or timid, puts in his or her two-cents worth, followed by an open star discussion, and ending with center pivot to reach closure if a "sense of the group" is desired.

Another common mix is pivot and star. Parliamentary procedure provides a formal control to keep the process from being subverted, but it is imposed as little as necessary. At each new topic, the rules are suspended to permit open discussion. If one or a few begin to dominate, the chair reasserts direct control. Other center pivot interventions are made to get a digression back on track, to reach closure, and to "move the agenda."

To keep your own options open, you may set ground rules that call for inputs and discussion but no "sense of the group" closures. When a group jells on a specific recommendation, members expect you to follow it even if the group is officially only "advisory." If you don't their noses get out of joint.

How Structured?

The structure of a group may be low, standard, or high. The most common informant group approach is "standard": critical discussion of items on a presented agenda, typically with a star-pivot mix. Star tends to be more dominant in advisory roles, pivot in authority-decision bodies.

Low structure encourages openness and creativity. In a standard discussion, many members, for fear of criticism or looking foolish, are reluctant to volunteer a new idea. It is safer to react than to initiate. The challenge is how to overcome their "fear of flying." In the 1950s, advertising man George Osborne invented a creative gimmick called brainstorming. Its ground rules are to suspend all critical judgments and just free-wheel wherever your creative imagination takes you. There are no limits. Ideas can be wild or "off the wall." No one criticizes another's ideas, but you can "hitchhike" on a previous idea; that is, carry it further or come up with a variation that it triggered in your mind. Everything is recorded unselectively. After the meeting, a staff person sifts out the promising ideas and collates them for the planner/decisionmaker, who may take it from there in a more traditional process.

The advantage of this is its open-ended freedom, creativity, and fun. A liability is inefficiency. For every good input you have to sift through a dozen worthless ones.

A *rigid structure* approach is the Nominal Group Technique (NGT) (Delbecq and Van de Ven, 1971; Delbecq et al., 1975), a strict feed-the-kitty style. It was developed to get maximum unhindered input, especially from those who may be ignored or underrepresented in normal planning. Recommended NGT size is six to ten. A larger group takes longer and is more tedious. The process is simple and orderly:

- Distribute a 5×7 card to each member.
- Define the subject, such as identifying needs or figuring out the best way to pursue an objective, and what inputs are wanted from the group.
- Allow thirty minutes for individuals to think and write their five most important inputs. Sometimes they are asked to rank their inputs from most to least important.
- Do a round robin in sequence, feeding each one's first ante into the kitty. No comments are permitted other than to identify "me too" if you had the same idea written down. Write each item on a flip chart. Add a check mark to an item for each "me too."
- When the first round is completed, repeat through five rounds until all written-down ideas are in the kitty.
- Distribute to each member a 3×5 card on which to vote for the five most important items on the flip chart. There may be a few minutes of open discussion before the vote, or none at all.
- The planner records the vote and takes the group recommendations on up to higher decision makers for that plan.

The greatest advantage of such a structured group is to equalize participation, preventing anyone from dominating other members. It is especially useful where members are unequal in status, power, confidence, quickness, or assertiveness. Because the ideas are developed before anyone speaks, and all ideas are laid out and collated before anyone can respond to them, it is an antidote to the tendency for the first ideas expressed to steer the group's attention.

The strength of a structured group is also its weakness. Equality is gained at the expense of give-and-take spontaneity. It is frustrating to be stimulated by another's idea with no opportunity to pick up on it in the meeting. There is no place for creative development and fine tuning of ideas. It can be boring to spend two hours listening passively to what you could have read and responded to in a fraction of the time.

Given the low level of interaction, might not more be achieved through interviews and dialogue with the individuals separately? Often, but not always. One reason to use a group could be that the participants would not talk freely on their own to an interviewer. In many organizations and settings, especially authoritarian and bureaucratic ones, staff and clients have nothing to gain and much to lose by speaking freely. NGT, with its precise, depersonalized formal procedures, is a safer setting in which to share knowledge and ideas.

Another reason to use the group may be organizational development. Bringing together a mixed staff group may increase their sense of belonging to the whole organization, not just their own pieces of the action. Even a mediocre NGT is an opportunity to get to know interdisciplinary peers better. For best results, hold it in a retreat setting with a nice luncheon before, and a social hour afterward.

COMMUNITY FORUM

Community forums have been advocated as a major needs assessment approach. A forum is not strictly a group but rather an *aggregation*, "a collection into an unorganized whole." It is an open public meeting which anyone may attend.

It has clear advantages. By being open to all on a self-selected basis, it reaches otherwise untapped sources and coincides with grassroots self-determination values. It has potential for insights, especially subjective and impressionistic ones, which complement the impersonal statistics of available data, the limited perspectives of traditional key informants, and the preselected multiple choices offered in a survey questionnaire. As a bonus, it attracts people with above-average interest who may be prospects for other involvements or follow-ups.

It also has flaws. It is too large and diverse for effective participation by most of the persons there. It is not representative. Average citizens rarely attend, and if they do, they may be timid about speaking out.

Forums are easily subverted. They attract people with an ax to grind which may be hostile to the plan or completely off the subject. Such people have no commitment to the purpose of the forum. It is an opportunity to beat their own drum. They may organize in advance and "stack" the audience. These participants may disrupt the agenda, drown out others who attempt to speak, create disturbances. This is exacerbated if the general attendance is low and indifferent.

Finally, whatever your formal disclaimers, holding a public forum can heighten expectations prematurely, creating a backlash when they are not met.

Among one's most useful informants are indigenous leaders and advocates. However, they often operate on two levels, an ideological public position and a private pragmatic realism about achieving limited gains. In the forum, what they say will be tailored to their public audience, not the planner. In individual interviews or small ad hoc groups with trusted fellow leaders, their not-for-attribution inputs may be far more useful. Further, in a forum, the ambience is often adversary, whereas the other settings are designed to create a collaborative atmosphere.

Community forums should be used sparingly. A series of small grassroots and specialized ad hoc informant groups is likely to give more insight at less risk to the planners. Where a forum is appropriate, as in public planning that must be open to input from all affected citizens, a structured hearing format may be preferable to an open style. All comments are addressed to the dais. Speakers must be recognized by the chair, who can limit domination by any individual or group. A typical rule is that no one can speak a second time if there is a first-time speaker asking to be recognized. Expectation may still be stirred up, but ironically this is less of a problem for hearings held by public bodies, thanks to cynical pessimism about their usual level of responsiveness.

SURVEY

Surveys obtain direct information from the target population. They require high technical competence in classical social research and statistics. If you are not expert, "hire it done" by a pro.

Face, Phone, or Mail?

Survey information may be obtained through *face-to-face* interviews, *telephone* interviews, or *mailed* questionnaires.

There is a major cost difference. Face-to-face is the most expensive, requiring staff time in each interview *plus* travel time and cost. If a repeat visit is needed to catch absent informants, the cost doubles. Phoning still requires the interview time, but eliminates the travel time and cost. Mailed questionnaires eliminate the staff interviewing costs altogether.

Theoretically one could survey the whole "universe," all persons within your defined population boundaries. For instance, in a medical school assessment, all 150 fourth-year students were polled. When the universe gets much larger than that, to interview them all becomes prohibitive.

Almost as reliable, and less costly, is a random "scientific" sample drawn to represent a cross section. This permits statistical projections to the entire population, give or take some leeway for random variations in the sample. The larger the sample, the smaller the leeway ("margin of error").

Some mailed questionnaires, especially from a prestigious sponsor to a highly educated and motivated constituency, have high response rates. For example, a dissertation survey of local pastors was mailed by a National Council of Churches executive who explained its importance and how he would use the information. It received an initial response rate of 80 percent, which rose to 90 percent with a follow-up reminder. Had it been mailed by the obscure doctoral student, a 25 percent response might have been predicted.

Unfortunately, mailed questionnaires generally have the lowest response rate of return of any survey method. You can disregard this if you assume that nonresponse is random and therefore that those answering are representative of the whole sample. However, it is more likely that the nonresponse is due to different characteristics from respondents. Thus, the lower the response rate, the less reliably can they be projected to the whole population.

A partial corrective to nonrespondent bias–at extra cost–is to do follow-up interviews with a sample of them to identify, and adjust for, the divergences.

Telephone interviews may have a built in sample bias. The famous Gallup Poll prediction that Dewey would defeat Truman solidly in 1948 was based on a "scientific" random sample of telephone numbers. In those days, many working class and poor people had no home phone. Thus a large segment of pro-Truman voters was left out.

Today most people have telephones, but the sample is distorted in another direction. It excludes those with unlisted numbers. Another biasing factor is answering machines and caller "ID" devices. Many people use them to screen out unwelcome intrusions into their privacy. Thus, independent and assertive people may be underrepresented.

Face-to-face personal interviewers are harder to reject, and "in the flesh" may be more trusted, leading to a higher response rate, especially with a policy of callbacks to people missed the first time. It is also the most expensive and complicated. For a majority of plans, it costs more than the gain in information may be worth, but it is excellent for a major project using comprehensive rational analysis. Even so, it has its flaws. It tends to underrepresent job moonlighters and single persons because they are hard to find at home.

Another angle on survey method is which generates the best answers? Are the questions understood and the answers clear? Face-to-face and phone interviewers can probe to clarify, but the questionnaire is rigid.

Is the respondent telling the truth? One school of thought says it is hardest to lie to a person's face, easier to lie to a voice on the phone, and easiest of all on an anonymous questionnaire. A contrary view claims that questionnaires are the most truthful because they are anonymous, and there is no need to cover up things that you would be embarrassed to tell someone face-to-face. The disembodied telephone voice falls in between. Perhaps it varies with the interviewer. In several areas of activity, I have been able to draw out more frank and complete information over the phone than through any other medium.

Pros and Cons

The key advantage of a survey is getting information direct from the horse's mouth. No one else may really know the felt needs and experiences of the targets. This neatly supplements data from statistical indicators and the varied perspectives of the key informants. Although there is no two-way dialogue or feedback, getting such broad grassroots input enhances self-determination.

In addition to the information itself, a sound survey tends to impress funders and public officials with the caliber of the planners and the presumed accuracy of their assessment.

On a broader but less intense scale, a poll does for the grassroots what key informant methods do for providers and actors: consciousness raising. In a health survey of low income persons, asking questions about a list of conditions made some respondents aware for the first time of problems they had accepted as normal and inevitable. From questions about which of a list of available health services they had used, many discovered for the first time where they could get help. Thus, a byproduct of the survey was an immediate increase in demand.

The limitations are well known. Number one is time and cost: is the benefit of a survey worth it?

Close behind is human fallibility, which inevitably results in *some* imperfections in methodology and technique. This leaves surveys vulnerable to pseudoprecision, where precise statistics are derived from imprecise samples, unwittingly slanted questions, and/or subtle differences among interviewers. If they are minor, take it into account and go on. If major, you have an expensive white elephant.

Nonscientific Surveys

Is there a shortcut? Let us assume that you would ideally like a scientific survey but lack the time, resources, or inclination. How about a survey that reaches out without rigorous sampling, such as the person who stands on a busy mall corridor and haphazardly buttonholes passersby with a marketing survey? Is a "quick and dirty" survey viable without meticulous sampling, obsession with wording, rigorous pretesting, etc.? The purist answer is "no" because it can mislead. Do it right or not at all.

As a pragmatist, I say go ahead *but do not process it as a survey with sophisticated statistics.* Call it "exploratory" and treat it as you would key informants, experienced intuition, and other "non-scientific methods" discussed in the chapter on reasoning.

HOW STRUCTURED?

In regard to both key informant interviews and surveys, there are pros and cons on how structured versus open-ended they should be.

Structured instruments have the huge asset that all responses are consistent, comparable, and able to be tabulated statistically. Every person is asked, so far as is humanly possible, the same questions in the same words and sequence with the same manner. They are easy to administer and analyze, for they are limited to short questions and a restricted choice of predetermined multiple choice, checklist, and true-false answers.

The price of precision is reductionism. You get answers only to what you ask and the choice of answers you permit, which means you miss any information you failed to anticipate in advance.

Sophisticated and insightful thinkers have a problem with black-and-white questions about their world, which is in technicolor with an infinite range of colors and shades. An accurate answer is "A in this aspect, C in that regard, B in such and such a situation, and none of the above if . . . ." Such informants face a Catch 22. They cannot avoid a misleading response. They must either select an untrue response or leave it blank. The latter is usually recorded as "don't know" or "no opinion," which could not be further from the truth.

Another problem is ambiguity. "It was a dark and rainy night". . . when I was visiting my parents in an unfamiliar place with narrow, winding dirt roads. My father said, "turn right here." Peering through the blurry windshield, I saw a dirt road on the left and immediately made a "turn, right here"–into the county dump.

"No," he cried, "I meant "turn right, here," pointing to a paved road a hundred yards ahead. Although researchers work hard to avoid this, they cannot completely avoid some "turn right here" misunderstandings.

An extreme *open-ended* interview might start with "well, how's the world going?" and let the respondent take it from there.

There are middle grounds, where you can get the best of both worlds. On a questionnaire, develop the standard short-answer questions. Group them into subject-related clusters. At the end of each cluster, add a space headed "comment." At the end of the questionnaire, add a page entitled, "any other comments?" For an interview schedule, the interviewer asks the direct questions first, then invites further comment.

After the short answers have been tabulated, record the comments separately as qualitative data. These answers can't be tabulated statistically, but they may provide rich insights, nuances, and anecdotes that can help the plan, as well as being quoted selectively to add human interest to the statistical report.

A needs assessment was prepared for what turned out to be the first statewide family court system, which would permit divorce for "incompatibility" but only after mandatory conciliation. A judge's added comment, quoted in the report, became the pro-family meeting ground of advocates and erstwhile opponents of the court reform act: "I have never presided over the death of a marriage, but I have conducted hundreds of funerals."

A structured key interview might be incrementally loosened. At its tightest, the interviewer reads the questions and writes the multiple choice response. A first loosening-up increment might be to ask the questions in order, but leave the responses open-ended rather than multiple choice. Go a little further, and you become flexible enough to permit the informant to pursue the question into related information and implications. A third loosening step is to give the informant a list of questions with permission to address them in the order he or she prefers.

If you want to do a genuine minimum-structure interview, prepare in advance a list of the areas to cover and kinds of information wanted, but play the interview itself by ear. Tell the informant what the needs assessment is for and draw him or her into discussion, perhaps with a general question or a simple pump primer. Once the respondent gets going, you may probe for further elaboration, variations, applications, etc. It is seemingly nonbounded, but you have a road map. If the respondent's first comment fits your #7 on your checklist, record it there, followed perhaps by comments recorded under your #2, #5, #8, and #2 again. Approaching closure, steer the discussion with timely questions to be sure that all the bases have been touched (in any order).

As with questionnaires, the more structured the interview, the more you can record in comparative and statistical ways. As you loosen up, you may still keep a few structured questions for which you want categorical responses, while the bulk has become prime "nonscientific" raw material.

HOW MUCH NEEDS ASSESSMENT?

> Do not merely listen to the word and deceive yourself.
> Do what it says.
>
> *—James 1:22*

Keep needs assessment in perspective. It is not sacred. It is a *means, not an end.* Its purpose is to *meet* needs: find out what they are and create a provision that will be used effectively.

Do only what you will use. "Use" refers to any and all functions suggested in Chapter 13 including, but rarely limited to, information.

Subject the needs assessment itself to cost and benefit analysis. Realistically, you are limited to what you can afford. In addition to budget, be sure to include indirect costs, such as staff time diverted from existing services or production. If what you can afford is less than ideal, do the best you can with what you have. Weak headlights are not as good as bright ones, but they are a big jump up from driving blind.

You may not spend all you can afford. Following the law of diminishing returns ("marginal utility"), weigh the cost of more NA against gain to your planning. Up to a point, improved planning is unquestionably worth the cost of the NA. As your information increases, the cost of getting more becomes steeper (for instance, an expensive survey), while the extra knowledge only marginally improves your decision making. The limit of NA is not when it ceases to contribute but rather when what it contributes is no longer worth the cost.

A related factor is the time available for NA. There have been some beautiful needs assessment studies that look impressive on the shelf but are failures, because the practical decision makers could not wait and acted without them. Plan your NA for the realistic time frame. The methods you use and the extensiveness with which they are applied must be doable in time you have.

Whatever needs assessment you do:

- Design it to provide as many bonus multifunction payoffs as possible.
- Recognize the results as imperfect contributions to the decision, which will ultimately be filtered through professional judgment, common sense, intuition, and practical politics. Use multiple methods and diverse sources within each method.
- Evaluate, in retrospect, its effectiveness and deficiencies to gain insight for future needs assessments. What good did it do? How did it improve the planning? How well did it perform its non-information functions? Were there unplanned side effects: good ones to build into future projects, bad ones to avoid next time?

When all is said and done, finish saying and start doing.

REFERENCES

Consumer's Union (1994). "Public interest pretenders." *Consumer Report's,* May, pp. 316-320.

Dalky, N. (1967). *Delphi.* Santa Monica: Rand.

Delbecq, A. and Van de Ven, A. (1971). "A group process model for problem identification." *Journal of Applied Behavioral Science,* 7, pp. 466-492.

Delbecq, A. et al. (1975). *"Group techniques for program planning: A guide to nominal group and delphi processes. "* Glenview: Scott Foresman.

Warheit, G., Bell, R., and Schwab, J. (1977). *Needs assessment approaches: Concepts and methods.* U.S. Govt, DHEW Publication #(ADM)77-472.

V. QUANTITATIVE PLANNING METHODS

Quantitative analysis dominates mainstream planning theory and practice, often to the point of ignoring what cannot be counted. It has always been central in physical, economic, and corporate planning, and it has become a major aspect of social and human service planning as well. Because of its ability to measure and compare diverse items on a consistent common denominator, it should be used with whatever lends itself to being counted, even in simple plans.

Chapter 15 summarizes the basic elements of quantitative analysis, and some methods of converting intangibles to numbers.

Chapter 16 goes the next step of reducing all good and bad things to economic numbers (dollars) as the universal measure of value. It progresses from its utilitarianism roots, through the classical liberalism of Pareto's "someone gains; nobody loses," to legitimizing harmful actions on condition that the victim is paid money as compensation, and ultimately to welfare economics, in which "good" or "bad" is reduced to aggregate dollar gains or losses for the collective economy.

The keystone of all economic planning models is assigning a dollar number to *everything*. Chapter 17 discusses a range of pricing techniques, plus how to adjust for a discrepancy between theory and reality: the fact that the "real" value (utility) of a dollar is not constant from person-to-person or year-to-year.

Chapter 18 is "where the rubber meets the road," numerical comparisons of gains (positive results) and costs (inputs plus losses suffered by anyone). It explains the distinction between three versions of this analysis: cost effectiveness, cost utility, and cost benefit.

These techniques can be valid, within their limitations, in analyzing inputs and results which have already taken place. However, all plans are for the future, which is uncertain. Chapter 19 describes a decision analysis method to predict the effect of uncontrolled factors on the probability of success and compute the "average" value of alternative action choices.

In each of the chapters in this section, an implicit dialectic is used, presenting the method positively, its limitations, how to mitigate its negatives and fill its gaps, and when to use or not use it.

Chapter 15

Painting by Numbers

Count: to have numerical value; importance; be worth considering.

No-account: of no consequence or importance.

Quantitative analysis is the cornerstone of traditional planning and finds its way to some degree into all planning.

- A *quantity* is "that property of anything which can be determined by mathematical measurement."
- To *measure* is "to ascertain the extent, dimensions, quantity, etc., of something, especially by comparison with a standard."
- *Tangible* is "having actual material form and substance; capable of being touched; able to be appraised for value."
- *Intangible* is "not easily defined, formulated or grasped." It cannot itself be mathematically measured.

INTERVAL MEASURES

To do valid quantitative analysis, measurements must be constant. This requires an *interval scale*, in which each number always has the same value in relation to every other number. The one we all know best is *arithmetic* progression, in which there is the same distance between each number. For instance, the difference between 2 and 3 must always be the same–and identical to the distance between 3 and 4. Ratio scales, such as logarithms and decibels in which each number is ten times its predecessor, are derived from it. Because of this constancy, the numbers can be related by adding, subtracting, multiplying, or dividing.

In quantitative analysis, we compare different items on the same property, by defining a common numerical measurement unit which is the same for all items at all times. This is relatively easy for physical measurements, where the unit may be calibrated to a standard gram or foot. It is more difficult to devise a fixed, invariable unit of measurement for such intangibles as general well being, happiness, emotional adjustment, and esthetics. Economics uses dollars (or £ or ¥) as the common denominator for comparing almost everything.

NOMINAL CATEGORIES

Data can instead be sorted by nominal ("name") categories based on some property (red or green, female or male, employed or not employed). Normally, only simple calculations can be made: the number of cases within each category, percentage distribution of cases among categories, or the one with the most cases (mode).

This is useful for planning where all you need are simple, crude measures such as breaking down methods of vacation travel into airplane, bus, automobile, or "other." It is also a practical compromise when dealing with things that can't be precisely measured either directly or indirectly via reliable indicators. This is often the case in human services and social planning. "There is more to be said for rough estimates of the precise concept than precise estimates of irrelevant concepts" (Mishan, 1976, p. 320).

Converting Nominal to Interval

By using only two mutually exclusive categories, "yes" and "no" (adopted or not, dry for six months or drinking again, employed or jobless), nominal data can be converted to interval numbers: yes = 1, no = 0. This can distinguish success ("1"), but it can't distinguish *how* successful. Since real life is seldom all or nothing, this method must draw an arbitrary line, above which is a full 1 and below which is an absolute 0. A job is a job, regardless of differences in wages or working conditions. In some planning, that is the best we can do.

ORDINAL SCALES

The ordinal scale *ranks* items in relation to such characteristics as desirability, feasibility, importance of need, or cost. This is one-dimensional: items can be ranked only on one thing at a time. (If you want to compare items on several aspects at once, you first develop a scale for each one and then combine them into a single, composite, weighted index scale.)

A standard process to develop the scale is paired comparisons. If A is higher than B, it is also higher than everything B outranks.

The bad news is that ordinal numbers are not constant in either value or intervals. They are relative. The key question is "compared to what?" The same performance might rank a student tenth in a super-bright honors class, but first in a poor class (which a colleague called being "the cream of the crap").

Similarly, the distances between adjacent rank numbers vary. Let us say a set of scores are 97-89-88-87-86-85-66. Their ordinal numbers (ranks) are 1-7. There is an eight-point difference between 1 and 2, and a whopping nineteen between 6 and 7, yet only four points separate 2 and 6.

You cannot statistically add, subtract, multiply, divide, or figure averages on rankings. There is one legitimate statistic: the median, which is arrived at by counting halfway from top to bottom. In the 1 through 7 list above, #4 (87) is the median.

The good news is that you *can* determine priority, one of the most important aspects of planning. It is particularly valuable in dealing with intangibles and in applying experience-intuitive judgments. Ordinal ranking may be "the way to go" in sorting out VIBES, key result areas, and goals, especially at the global and strategic levels.

Ranking by Clusters

If the number of cases makes individual ranking cumbersome, you can revert to our planning standby process of operating by stages. First do a scan in which you assign cases into such broad-stroke categories as high, medium, and low.

Then rank the more manageable number of cases within each cluster. If ranking just by cluster is enough to serve your purpose or the data simply does not support making finer distinctions, you can dispense with the second stage.

A variation of this has a neutral midpoint from which both negative and positive categories diverge. On occasion, religions have even graded afterlife this way. One Eastern religion has nine levels of bliss (as in "I am on cloud nine"). Dante's inferno had nine levels of hell, each worse than the one before. Put these together and you have categories ranked from –9 to +9 (with a midpoint 0 for Dante's limbo, in which souls drift around aimlessly with neither pleasure nor pain).

In my college, we had a five-point positive-negative grading scale, requiring a midpoint C-average to remain enrolled. Above C was distinction. Below C was extinction. We referred to the lower two clusters as "Death Valley grades: below sea [C] level."

Using Invalid Statistics with Ordinal Numbers

Is it ever all right to do any statistics with ordinal rankings of individual cases or clusters? Let's look at it dialectically.

The *thesis:* statistics are not valid if the numbers are not interval. Period! If you have a sow's ear, you can't make a silk purse from it even with the best needlework skills.

The *antithesis:* that is technically true, but "everybody does it" anyhow. Take the GPA. It is statistically invalid, among other reasons, because the cluster rankings have unequal intervals. In my graduate program, the distance between A (4) and B (3), both of which are fully satisfactory, is less than the distance between B and substandard-pass C (2). There is a still greater distance between C and D (1), which automatically flunks the student out of the program. All of our university administrators have studied advanced statistics, yet from these ordinal rankings they calculate averages to 0.01 of a point on the transcript and use that decimal number as the primary basis for academic awards (a classic example of pseudoprecision). When challenged, their answers are, "This is how we have always done it" and "We don't have anything better." Well if all those PhDs do it, why shouldn't we peasants do it too!

A *synthesis* is to do it where it's useful for insights, being careful to avoid any claims, to ourselves or others, of scientific or technical validity. Coyle (1972, p. 83) refers to "the art of giving bad answers to questions to which otherwise worse answers would be given." For instance, although we find conventional GPA unreliable for differentiating between a 3.39 and a 3.43 student, we might use it to get rough approximations. For example, my department sets 3 (or alternative evidence of current academic ability) as a normal minimum standard to be reviewed for possible admission to a program in which the current students had an average undergraduate GPA of 3.5.

UNDER THE STREETLIGHT: QUANTIFYING THROUGH INDICATORS

> Mutt finds Jeff on his hands and knees under a corner street-light. Jeff explains he has lost a five dollar bill. Mutt helps search. After scouring the area, he asks Jeff, "Are you sure you lost it here?" "No, I lost it up there [pointing to the dark middle of the block] but the light is better here."
>
> —"Mutt and Jeff" *comic strip*

If you can't measure a qualitative element, is there something nearby which you *can* measure? *Indicate* means "to show; point to; give sign and token of." In planning, an indicator is a quantitative property which represents an unmeasurable entity. The extent of the real thing is *inferred* from the indicator. Schools use reading test scores as indicators of actual reading ability. Economists use income as an indicator of well-being. Scores on standardized knowledge tests are used by licensing boards as indicators of professional competence and skill. Body temperature is used as an indicator of infection.

An indicator needs two things to be useful. One is that its numbers are interval and measurements consistent.

The other is *correlation.* An indicator is *valid* to the extent that it accurately represents the real thing. A test may be a valid measure of short-term knowledge but an invalid indicator of true education ("development of the special and general abilities of the mind").

Pragmatically, we recognize that it is nearly impossible to have perfect correlation between a qualitative entity and its numerical indicator. We accept it within tolerable limits. What is a tolerable limit: ±10 percent, ±20 percent? There is no set guideline. How could you ever be sure, since the reason for the indicator in the first place is inability to measure the entity itself precisely? We have to use our best judgment on whether the imperfect indicator is better than none. Many are. Some are not: an inaccurate indicator that misdirects planning might be worse than none at all.

An indicator is *reliable* to the extent that it *varies at the same rate* as the entity. Every valid indicator is also reliable. Invalid measures may sometimes be reliable anyway. My humidity gauge is always wrong. It reads 90 when the humidity is 75, and 65 when it is 50. However, it is reliable, for it varies consistently with the real humidity, which is always fifteen points lower than the reading.

Sometimes an indicator may be unreliable in certain circumstances but useful selectively. The Miller's Analogy Test (MAT) is designed to measure analogical reasoning skills. Its questions are premised on the common experience and vocabulary pool of a mainstream middle-class American culture. For persons who have this background, test scores seem to be a fairly reliable indicator. However, foreign students, those with English as a second language, and persons from nonmainstream American cultures don't have the assumed experiences and vocabulary. For them, the MAT score is by no means a reliable indicator of *reasoning ability.*

While, in principle indicators should be as precisely valid as possible, remember that they are only tools, not ends in themselves. Why go to the trouble reaching for a level of precision you don't need. For instance, the transcripts of all graduates of one very selective and demanding doctoral program carry only the grade of S (Satisfactory) for each course and dissertation.

Pitfalls of Indicators

A common pitfall is to *reify* ("to treat an abstraction as a concrete material object") the indicator as if it were the element itself. Indicators inherently correlate only imperfectly, and they are reductionist, reducing a complex quality to a number. As discussed, this is okay as long as you take its limitations into account in your use of it. Regretfully, it is common to present a statistical analysis of the indicator as if it were the real thing. To do so is arrogant (excessive claims to expert knowledge), lazy (avoiding inconvenience), or dumb (unaware of the discrepancy).

A planning fallout of this is *goal displacement*. Initially, our goal relates to the entity. We know that and use it properly. After a while we get used to the indicator and begin to treat it, consciously or not, as if it were the actual entity. Rewards and actions are based on indicator scores. People aren't stupid. If the rewards are based on the indicator, they displace the goal onto the indicator.

For example, years ago New York State achieved higher educational performance than other states by using standardized statewide Board of Regents tests as indicators of school and student performance. The aim was to identify and upgrade deficient programs. This worked, up to a point. However, by the time I was in high school, the exam had displaced education as the goal. The last quarter of each course was spent being drilled over and over for it, including practicing on more than a dozen of the previously-administered exams, to raise our scores on "the Regents." All new learning and rational development came to a standstill. Thus the indicator displaced the education as a goal, resulting in a 25 percent reduction of what it was intended to accomplish.

Using Indicators

Indicators can and should be used where feasible, to take advantage of the many opportunities which quantification permits. To be effective, they should meet the following criteria:

- A clearly defined real objective or entity.
- Careful selection and continuous review of the indicator to be sure it is accurate enough to meet the planner's requirements.
- Alertness to intervening variables that weaken its reliability, and where possible, incorporating such variables into a revised indicator.
- Application only within its limits, which are acknowledged openly.

- Used within a multibased analysis, which will probably include some "pure" quantitative data, other indicators, and "nonscientific methods."
- Monitoring for goal displacement, and corrections to get back on track.

GENERAL QUANTITATIVE PROS AND CONS

Numbers are an excellent aid to reasoning, but it's an increasingly common error to use only the numbers available and to fail to quantify the rest of the situation.

—Marilyn vos Savant, 1995

Advantages

Quantitative analysis measures inputs and outcomes: needs, effects, and resources to get the job done. It helps to define objectives and assess whether they were achieved. It disciplines evaluation, reducing the temptation (and ability) to fudge.

It helps to choose among alternatives by providing a common denominator for comparing them. It documents the nature and extent of the need, the probable cost of implementation, and the worth of doing it at all. It may be used to widen your perspective by estimating (in advance) and monitoring (after the fact) significant side effects.

Not to be ignored is that it impresses others, especially sponsors, authorities, and funders. "People tend to associate numbers with accuracy, exact numbers with certainty, and certainty with authority that is not subject to challenge" (Branch, 1990, p. 170).

Quantomania

The people were deeply troubled; that you well know, and they said to me, "Make us gods to go ahead of us."

—Aaron to Moses
Exodus 32:23

A liability of quantitative technology is that its very competence tends to *displace* other methods. "Powerful tools always change the processes to which they are introduced. In time, the entire activity is modified to suit what the new tools can and cannot do. . . . It is therefore proper to ask what the new servant will do to the master and the master's purpose" (Vickers, 1970, p. 103).

Carried to a logical extreme, "*quantomania*" is "a mathematical messiah that can quantify and analyze the entire output of a social organism" (Hughes and Mann, 1969). It is "a sacrifice of meaning on the altar of quantification in order to save face" (Mishan, 1976, p. 407).

The prospect is tempting. "Knowledge is hard to obtain; the mind of man is small and simple, while the world is large and complex. Hence the temptation to imply by a cover word possession of the very thing, causal knowledge, that is missing" (Wildavsky, 1973, pp. 141-42).

This "religion" has its own technocratic moral code. "The emphasis on scientific rigor in economics—where cost benefit analyses convert social and moral choices into pseudo-technical ones—is a reflection of the widespread belief that all problems have technical solution" (Rothman and Tooler, 1986, p. 8).

Close Your Eyes and Maybe It Will Go Away

Quantomania can provide a quasireligious defense against wicked problems by excommunicating them. This is what classical positivism and materialism do. Positivism is "a system of philosophy which is based solely on observable, scientific facts." Its cousin, materialism, is "the doctrine that everything in the world, including thought, will, and feeling, can be explained only in terms of matter." Modern science itself has refuted the longstanding atomism theory of solid matter, on which these philosophies were based. Nevertheless, mainstream quantitative planning still practices them, de facto.

Economic planning does not actually deny the existence of intangibles. It merely dismisses them as irrelevant or too low a priority to deal with. According to hard-nosed businesspeople, sooner or later it all comes down to a bottom line measured in dollars.

If all else fails, one can simply decide to avoid wicked problems, not because they aren't there but because it is too hard (or just inconvenient) to deal with them.

> To some extent, alleged omissions of considerations of "social merit" in specific cost benefit studies can be ascribed to the existing difficulties of evaluation. If the benefit of such "good" things as better health, improved education, expanded recreational facilities, etc. could be satisfactorily measured, the impact of an investment project in these things would indeed be incorporated into the cost benefit calculation. (Mishan, 1976, p. 405)

GIGO

> The Government are very keen on amassing statistics. They collect them, add them, raise them to the nth power, take the cube root, and prepare wonderful diagrams. But you must never forget that every one of these figures comes in the first instance from the village watchman, who just puts down what he damn pleases.

> —Sir Josiah Stamp, Inland Revenue Dept., ca. 1900

A common quantomania pitfall is pseudoprecision, precisely correct calculation of imprecise numbers. In computerese, this is referred to as GIGO (Garbage In → Garbage Out). In addition to measurement errors, inaccuracies occur to the extent that data is incomplete, indicators fall short of correlating with the real thing, and "guesstimates" miss the bullseye.

Quantification also has an inherent *programming* GIGO: its model is incomplete, leaving out key elements. The result may be "right" answers–to the wrong questions.

USING QUANTITATIVE ANALYSIS

> But who has ever produced anything approximately comprehensive for non-linear systems consisting of non-homogeneous parts?

> —Augustinovics, 1975

Because of its advantages, quantitative methods should be used for whatever lends itself to being counted. It is hard to imagine good corporate planning, physical planning, or national social and economic planning–or any complex plan–without it.

It is usually part of individual micro planning as well. In my house hunting, used to illustrate a simple needs assessment in Chapter 13, quantitative analysis played an important part. In selecting communities, after narrowing them down to a few choices through key informants, I collected commuter time data (via timetables) and percentage of high school graduates going on to college, to verify and compare the finalist communities. In order to set my price range, I had to (1) figure out the monthly payments I could afford (based on family income and expenditure records), and (2) calculate the maximum mortgage on which the monthly payment was affordable (based on interest rates, principle payoff rate, and escrows for taxes and insurance). The quantitative data were relatively simple and easy to obtain, but they were critical to the planning decisions.

When not to use it? It is not required for *every* situation. It is not necessary for planning some spiritual, aesthetic, and emotional goals.

Quantitative analysis is a tool, not a divine revelation. It needs to be used with a *soupçon* of humility, claiming only what the model, the indicators, and the measuring instruments can justify. This avoids mistakes caused by overreaching. It also increases your credibility. As Abraham Lincoln said, "You can fool some of the people all of the time, and all of the people some of the time, but you cannot fool all of the people all of the time."

> If the unmeasurable effect is completely beyond his range of reasonable guesses, so that the decision cannot be reached . . . on the basis of the measurable data . . . he serves the public better by confessing the truth. . . . Although the economist is unable to place a valuation on some critical magnitude he should provide the public with whatever about it that he has (including informed guesses on any aspect of it). (Mishan, 1976, pp. 407-408)

Don't choose between quantitative and qualitative. "This do without neglecting the other." Quantitative analysis is most effective as part of a multidimensional approach, along with qualitative data and the nonscience rational methods. Such planning is synoptic, "affording or taking a general view of the whole or of the principal parts of a subject."

REFERENCES

Augustinovics, M. (1975). "Integration of mathematics and traditional methods of planning." In Bornstein, M., *Economic planning: East and West.* Cambridge, MA: Ballinger, p. 138.

Branch, M. (1990). *Planning: A universal process.* New York: Praeger.

Coyle, R. (1972). *Decision Analysis.* London: Nelson.

Hughes, J. and Mann, L. (1969). "Systems and planning theory." *Journal of the American Institute of Planners*, 35, pp. 330-333.

Mishan, E. (1976). *Cost-benefit analysis.* 2nd ed. New York: Praeger.

Rothman, J. and Tooler, M. (1986). "Planning theory and planning practice: Roles and attitudes of planners." In Dluhy, M. and Chen, K. (Eds.), *Interdisciplinary planning.* New York: Center for Urban Planning.

Savant, M. vos (1995). "Ask Marilyn." *Parade*, April 23, 1995.

Vickers, G. (1970). *Value systems and social progress.* Baltimore: Penguin.

Wildavsky, A. (1973). "If planning is everything, maybe it's nothing." *Policy Sciences*, 4, pp. 127-153.

Chapter 16

By Bread Alone:
Economic Planning Models

Things are in the saddle and ride mankind.

–Ralph Waldo Emerson

Economic models dominate large-scale planning. To understand their assets and their limitations, we need to see "where they are coming from."

THE FOUNDATION: UTILITARIANISM

In 1789, moral philosopher Jeremy Bentham came up with *utilitarianism*, which the dictionary defines as "the ethical doctrine that virtue is based on *utility* and that conduct should be directed toward promoting the greatest happiness for the greatest number." To make this manageable, Bentham reduced happiness and unhappiness to the concrete experiences of pleasure and pain by individuals. For net utility, subtract the pain caused from the pleasure gained. He developed guidelines for measuring:

- *Duration:* how long it lasts.
- *Intensity:* how strongly it is felt.
- *Probability:* how certain or uncertain the results are.
- *Propinquity:* how immediate the gratification.
- *Extent:* how many persons affected.

REDUCTION TO ECONOMIC UTILITY

You *can* buy happiness.

The problem is figuring out how to put numbers on such intangibles so that they can be scored and processed mathematically. This requires a widely accepted single *common denominator* for measuring and comparing everything.

Economics found the solution. First it reduced utility from "happiness" to "satisfaction of a human want or need." Then it restricted "satisfaction" to *commodities*, "things which can be bought and sold." The next logical step was to substitute purchasing power, the ability to buy them, for the commodities themselves. A sign of this process can be seen in the shift from the Declaration of Independence's "life, liberty, and the pursuit of *happiness*" to the Fourteenth Amendment's "life, liberty, or *property*" a century later. The bottom line: happiness is measured by the value of property.

In economic utility, money is the ultimate value to which all other values must be converted, or they cannot be entered into the equation. Thus, an injury on the job is measured not in relation to the worker's pain or quality of life but as a purely economic loss—to the employer, the worker, the insurance company, and/or the taxpayer. Using this criterion in the 1980s, occupational safety and health standards were enforced only when the money to be saved by preventing injury exceeded the cost of the safety measure.

Advantages

The advantages of economic utility are neatness and universality. By reducing everything to a single dimension, it can analyze vast amounts of data. It can compare all costs and all effects of all goods and services. It can even bring some intangible values into the equation by converting them to dollar equivalents. This makes almost everything in the world negotiable, compensable, and exchangeable.

This makes sense. Money has been used as a universal common denominator of value for more than 5,000 years. Cattle were the common denominator of value. Later, for convenience, metal pictures of cattle enabled ownership to change without moving the real animal each time. This evolved into general coins and precious metals as common tender with standard exchange values. Their big advantage was wide acceptance and portability. We progressed to still more portable and convenient paper money that represented the heavier gold or silver coins. Electronic transfers carried this to its logical extreme, where nothing physical at all changes hands.

When economic utility is criticized for its flaws, the response is, "Okay, fine. What will we use instead?" Is there any other way to make *optimizing* choices; that is, to select the course of action with the best payoff? Can we even function without such a universal denominator?

Limitations

The primary strength of economic utility is also its greatest limitation: reductionism. It squeezes data into one dimension to fit its single tool, subordinating all other social, cultural, spiritual, aesthetic, and emotional dimensions of life. The virtues of the economic planning model may be subverted by *overreaching*. Warns Peter Self (1975, pp. 7-9):

> Econocrats attempt to turn economics into a master science of human values, capable of disclosing and quantifying these values according to some "objective" criterion of value known to economists. . . . Has the economist got any genuine yardstick for measuring objectively a diversity of factors other than the very limited criterion provided by market prices or other forms of financial data? . . . . If he has not, then the result may be less, not more, rational than would be a primarily qualitative form of analysis, because of the spurious appearance of reliability which a quantified set of data conveys.

Another limitation to be mindful of in applying the economic planning model is its foundation in the assumptions of classical economics about the human condition:

- *Pure self-interest.* "Man, it is assumed, pursues his self interest because of an acquisitive instinct or biological need."

- *"Economic man."* "Self interest is seen in economic terms; he acquires and consumes material goods; he avoids economic loss" (Wilensky and Lebeaux, 1965, p. 33).
- *Informed rational choice.* Mishan (1976, p. 309) observes wryly, "People's imperfect knowledge of economic opportunities, their imprudence and unworldliness, has never prevented economics from accepting as basic data the amounts people freely choose at given prices."
- *Free choice.* This assumes a free market which is not constrained by government policies, racism, classism, sexism, or anticompetitive monopolies.

Use It Selectively

In summary, the economic planning model can tell us much about many things, but it is never sufficient by itself, for "man does *not* live by bread alone." Within its legitimate sphere, it is irreplaceable. Use it as a key input to decision making, but stop short of making it the final authority.

Cynics say not to worry about its faults because it's a paper tiger. While economic utility is officially embraced by governments and corporations as their formal planning method, the "real" de facto decision makers (executives, boards, politicians, etc.) are only modestly influenced by these experts. They rarely read all the data. They are swayed more, for better or for worse, by vested interests, political expedience, their gut feelings, and the traditional culture of their society, party, organization, profession, or other reference groups.

WHATEVER HAPPENED TO PARETO'S IMPROVEMENT?

The Pareto Improvement

About 1897, Vilfredo Pareto developed a simple libertarian guideline for utilitarian decisions, known as the "Pareto Improvement." Any change is an "improvement" if someone is better off, and no one is worse off. When Princeton went coed, there was an outcry from its all-male alumni that women would usurp half of the slots available for the traditional constituency it had served for two centuries. The university's Pareto Improvement response was to enlarge the student body, which added females without loss to any male applicant.

The Economic Revision: Compensation

Later economists revised the Pareto Improvement to incorporate economic utility. The key premise is that utility is transitive, able to "go across." Any particular utility is exchangeable for another of equal value—or rather enough money to purchase something equivalent (i.e., *compensation*).

A key principle is *indemnity*, after-the-fact "payment or reimbursement for loss, damage, etc." Insurance and lawsuits operate on this principle. If your car or cargo is destroyed, you will get money to buy another one. If you die prematurely, your dependents receive money to replace your lost income.

Twentieth-century social planning took a giant step further, legitimizing *premeditated* harm to others, as long as compensation for that harm is also planned.

This violates the core liberty values of Locke, Jefferson, Mill, and Pareto, as well as the fundamental free market premise of a willing buyer and a willing seller. If planners condemn your home to make way for a new freeway, you are not a willing seller but the recipient of a Godfather "offer you can't refuse."

What else can the planner do? For the greater (aggregate) good we need that freeway. Would it not be unfair to deprive thousands of daily commuters because of your old house, which ain't so hot anyhow? What could be more fair?

This is an unresolvable dilemma. We don't have the moral right to harm, yet we have a moral obligation to do the good. Without the right to harm, no large-scale planning would be possible. In that context, the economic version of the Pareto Improvement offers a widely used "gray-area ethics" compromise.

Potential Pareto Improvement

The final revision (Welfare Economics, described below) adds a hook to the economic version of the Pareto Improvement. While the gains must be enough to cover compensation to the losers, that compensation need not actually be made.

WELFARE ECONOMICS:
AGGREGATE ECONOMIC UTILITY

It's bigger than the both of us.

*   *   *

The test of our progress is not whether we add more to the abundance of those who have much; it is whether we provide enough for those who have little.

—Franklin D. Roosevelt

Bentham reduced happiness to pleasures and pains. Economics reduced pleasure and pain to dollars (or lack thereof) which can buy desired commodities. It still referred to each individual.

Welfare economics (WE) made the next reduction by narrowing gain/loss considerations to the *aggregate* (from the Latin for "to lead a herd") without reference to what happens to any individual member of the herd. "Strict economic rationality means getting the most national income out of a given investment. The end is to increase the real GNP, no matter who receives it and the means is an investment expenditure, no matter who pays for it" (Wildavsky, 1973, p. 145).

In the second half of the twentieth century, welfare economics and its principle tool, cost-benefit analysis, became the prime economic model for most business and public planning, as well as many nonprofit human service programs.

Welfare economics is firmly rooted in the unitary-collective worldview and the biological organism system. The interest of the whole body transcends that of any of its parts. It makes central planning decisions to maximize the size of the pie without reference to internal distribution of the slices. Because of its indifference to the effects on individuals, WE is not utilitarian in the classic sense, for it does not concern itself with "the greatest good for the greatest *number.*"

Since it is not concerned with distribution, "fairness" concepts such as equality, equity, adequacy, and justice are irrelevant. A popular Depression song goes, "There's nothing surer, the rich get rich and the poor get poorer." This is desirable as long as the rich get rich faster than the poor get poorer.

Ironically, "welfare" economics has been used heavily as an *antiwelfare* rationale. There is often less profit in serving the aged, the ill, or the poor. Economist Mishan (1976, p. 394) objected, "It is not enough that the outcome of an ideal cost benefit analysis be positive. It must be shown, among other things, that the resulting distributional changes are not perceptibly regressive and that no gross inequities are perpetrated."

Some advocates argue that it does achieve the utilitarian goal automatically because of *Pareto's Law*, that the distribution of income is always essentially the same. Andrew Carnegie made the same assumption in his *Gospel of Wealth* (1900). Inequality exists, but it is constant. When business and investors prosper, the benefits will *trickle down* proportionately to the middle and lower classes. Thus, everyone benefits proportionally from any WE gain. Unfortunately, this is not always true. In the 1980s, American per capita income increased, but almost all of the gain went to the upper third, while the average income of wage-earner families went *down*.

Nevertheless, welfare economics is a useful input to macro economic, physical, and business planning by providing an aggregate overview. This may be particularly beneficial to a corporation whose parts (departments, employees, etc.) are explicitly subordinate to overall corporate interests.

It is more problematical for a government, which is legally and morally bound to provide "*equal* protection under the law" to every citizen. Even so, a general overview can be an invaluable check and balance against predatory interests who, in pursuit of their narrow gains, propose plans that would do more harm than good to the whole society. Astute environmentalists, for instance, frequently use it this way.

It may also add needed perspective to the loose cannon of disjointed muddling-through planning, which acts case by case without regard to larger consequences. There is the old story of the discount store owner whose prices really were "below cost," so that he lost money on each item sold. "How can you make a profit?" he was asked. "I make it up on volume." He could use a bit of aggregate perspective.

Using Welfare Economics

Centralized welfare economics data may be applied in different ways. The five levels below are based on Bicanic's typology of degrees of compulsion in government planning (1967, 42-46):

1. *Informative.* Provide the data as input to independent planners.
2. *Advisory.* As in market research, make nonbinding recommendations, backed by the data.
3. *Stimulative.* Based on the data, set central goals and provide carrot-and-stick incentives to implement them.
4. *Directive.* Set goals based on welfare economics analysis, and implement them directly or by delegation.
5. *Coercive.* Develop and impose a centrally determined plan with no regard to the interests of those involved or affected.

Welfare economics perspective can be used responsibly if the planner *also* is giving attention to:

- Distribution intents and effects.
- Who takes the loss/harm, and how.
- Provision of real (not just potential) compensation to harmed persons.
- A framework of explicit social values.
- The marginal utility factor (to be discussed in the next chapter).

REFERENCES

Bentham, J. (1823/1948). *An introduction to the principles of morals and legislation.* New York: Hafner.
Bicanic, R. (1967). *Problems of planning East and West.* Hague:Mouton.
Carnegie, A. (1900). *The gospel of wealth.* In *Introduction to contemporary civilization in the West,* Vol II. (1946). New York: Columbia University Press, pp. 617-631.

Mishan, E. (1976). *Cost-benefit analysis.* 2nd ed. New York: Praeger.
Self, P. (1975). *Econocrats and the policy process.* London: Macmillan.
Wildavsky, A. (1973). "If planning is everything, maybe it's nothing." *Policy Sciences*, 4, pp.127-153.
Wilensky, H. and Lebeaux, C. (1965). *Industrial society and social welfare.* 2nd ed. New York: Free Press.

Chapter 17

Everything Has Its Price

A man who knows the price of everything and the value of nothing.

—Oscar Wilde

Planning a trip, I took a night school course in Italian. The instructor said we needed to know only five words to get by as tourists: "Quanto costo in dollars?" and, whatever the response, "Troppo!" (too much). Economic planners can get by with the first four. (Their bosses often add the fifth.)

Price is "the amount of money for which anything is bought, sold, or offered for sale." Robert Walpole, an eighteenth-century English politician, observed of his colleagues, "All men have their price." The dominant planning model goes further: *everything* has its price.

The easiest and most common approach is *market* price, whatever is actually paid for a home, a sweater, or a day's work. It is simple, neat, and by definition avoids arguments: value is whatever was paid. No issues are raised about what a worker "really" deserves or the "true" value of a designer dress. By this measure, a tort lawyer is worth far more than a pastor who has as much or more training, works just as hard, and allegedly contributes much good to society. *Vox populi.* The people have voted with their pocketbooks for the lawyer.

So far, so good. But how do you price something that has not directly been bought and sold? Economists resort to *inferred* market pricing techniques, which estimate what someone *would* pay, or they resort to arbitrary valuation of intangibles.

ILLUSTRATION: PUTTING A PRICE ON DEATH

What price glory, Captain?

—Maxwell Anderson

Economic planning puts a dollar price on life itself. For example, in 1984, after Congress passed several laws to protect people by regulating environmental pollution, occupational safety and health, air traffic safety, etc., the U.S. Office of Management and Budget ordered enforcement agencies not to require correctives that cost more than the lives saved were worth. *The New York Times* reported, in an article entitled, "What is the Audited Value of Life?":

> The value of human life has eluded poets, theologians, and philosophers for centuries, but the Government has an answer. . . . In evaluating a new regulation, an agency will try to estimate how many lives it will save, what it will cost to adopt the rule, and thus the cost per life saved. This cost is weighed against the [dollar] value of those lives as part of the "regulatory impact analysis" demanded by the Reagan Administration. (Keller, 1984)

Gross Production

There are different ways to calculate the price of life. A traditional measure has been *gross production*. The process is a simple market approach which assumes that salary is a true measure of the value of a worker's contribution. The arithmetic is easy. Try it. To find out the value of your life, multiply your annual salary by the number of years remaining until age 65. (How do I explain to my wonderful spouse, who retired last year, that she is a no-'count wife?)

The basic premise is that economic production defines the value of a human life. There is no intrinsic right to life. There is no officially recognized value in noneconomic social contributions, intangible qualities of life, or intangible losses such as pain or bereavement.

This seems a bit arbitrary. Its effects are sexist, racist, ageist, and classist. Tying price to earning power means that upper-income lives are worth more than workers' lives. Women and minorities who have suffered discrimination and/or institutionalized inequalities average lower earnings than white males. Therefore, on the average, their lives are of less value.

Is this a sufficiently accurate pricing method to use as a basis for planning? What planning? By itself, its implicit value premises can lead to debatable social planning choices. For instance, in setting priorities for "universal" health coverage, Nobel economist Friedrich von Hayek (1960) applied the work-production yardstick faithfully when he urged, "It may seem harsh, but it is in the interests of all that, under [the British national health care] system, those with full earning capacity should often be rapidly cured . . . at the expense of some neglect of the aged . . . who will never again contribute to the [economic] needs of the rest." Carried to its logical conclusion, upon retirement should we not be given a gold watch and then sent to the gas chamber? (The watch, which still has value, can be recycled.)

On the other hand, in planning family security, can you think of a better basis for deciding how much life insurance to buy, or a homemaker's decision to go back to school to develop new earning power as an alternative life insurance policy?

Net Production

An economic criticism of the gross production measure is that not all of the worker's production is net contribution to "the economy." If you die, your lost production is offset by saving the cost of maintaining you. Therefore, the "real" value of your life is your *surplus* production: what you produce *minus* what you spend on yourself.

This raises a paradox: if this is a universal measure of the value of human life, then it applies to every person alive. If so, who is left to be "the economy" that will consume everyone's surplus production? Some of my colleagues have no problem answering this question. They say the whole point of capitalism is for owners to make a profit from the surplus production of labor. Thus, the true value of a worker is his or her surplus labor.

Risk Premium

Ideally, in classical economics the price of each individual's life is decided by that person. However, planners don't like this. With no consistent standard, the numbers do not qualify for quantitative analysis.

A compromise is to let people determine their worth through market transactions, particularly the price a person will accept to take on a risk. If a skyscraper construction worker has to be paid $5 per hour more than low-rise workers to take a job on which one person in a hundred is killed each year, his price (at 2,000 hours per year) is $10,000 for a 100-to-1 bet. To calculate the price at which he values his life, divide the premium by the probability of death: $10,000 ÷ 1/100 = $1,000,000.

Merkhofer (1986) cited studies in which this approach produced price tags of $400,000 to $7,000,000. The risk premium of life varied by occupation, with high-risk workers such as bartenders and firemen setting lower prices and white-collar workers predictably at the high end.

Such calculations are based on several a priori assumptions, for which empirical doubts may exist:

- Free choice between hazardous and safe jobs. Persons with higher education choose safer jobs because they have the choice. For less advantaged workers, on the other hand, the alternative is not lower income but none at all.
- The decision is based only on economic motive, whereas dangerous jobs may be chosen fully or in part because of family tradition, peer social pressure, prestige, and excitement.
- The average worker does a conscious rational analysis of reward versus risk. Did you? Many people, especially younger ones, have no sense of the reality of their own death. For them, a "risk premium" looks like a pure gain.
- Individuals' self-valuation is normative. If workers themselves place a low value on their lives, should society officially do likewise?

De Facto

The de facto value of life does not worry about what the price is based on. It simply asks what has actually been paid for deaths. A World War II combat soldier's life was worth $10,000, the amount of his GI life insurance. A commonly used measure is jury awards and other settlements of lawsuits. States which set ceilings on medical malpractice awards have, de facto, set the price of a life.

Is Life Priceless?

> The loss of honest and industrious men's lives cannot be valued at any price.
>
> *—Gov. William Bradford, Plymouth Plantation*

> We hold these truths to be self-evident, that all men are . . . endowed by their creator with certain unalienable rights, that among them are life . . . .
>
> *—Declaration of Independence*

> We believe the human person is sacred—the clearest reflection of God among us.
>
> *—National Council of Catholic Bishops*

If putting a dollar price on life goes against the professed values of American culture, why do we do it anyway? Those who do it argue that competing interests for limited resources is an unavoidable fact. Tradeoffs *will* be made one way or another. In large-scale planning it is impossible to deal individually with all cases, so quantitative methods *will* be used.

Even if life may be priceless, they say, putting a price on it is better than leaving it out of the planning equation altogether. Some deterrence and compensation is better than none, and within the system we can work incrementally closer to the "priceless" ideal by revising the pricing standard upward. Without the rational structure of pricing, we face a chaotic jungle in which there is no orderly basis for decision, regulation, or compromise. The half-a-loaf Occupational Safety and Health policies of the 1980s are preferable to the callous disregard of the value of life in Hitler's slave labor camps or in nineteenth-century factories.

PRICING TIME

Time is money.

—Benjamin Franklin

If you want to do cost-benefit analysis, all costs must be converted to dollars. A key cost is time.

The most common way to price time is an *analogous wage*. In strict nonprofit cost accounting, the cash equivalent value of a volunteer's time must be recorded as a budget expenditure to get a true cost effectiveness measure. Properly priced, it should be the price per hour paid for staff members with comparable skills and duties. Otherwise, the "real" cost of giving the service would be understated and not comparable with other programs. (The income budget then shows that cash value as a contribution from the volunteer.)

This method was also proposed as a corrective to the undervaluing a homemaker. Cash out her time value. Initially the analogous paid employment standard was that of a charwoman, which reflected the economists' perception of "women's work." Women countered by itemizing and pricing activities for which the analogous paid employment is professional and administrative.

Analogous wage is also used in computing the value of leisure time. In a cost-benefit study for a proposed commuter line which would cut thirty minutes each way from commuting, planners computed the value of travel time saved at the commuters' average wage level ($20 per hour). One hour for each of 200 commuting days @ $20 equals $4,000 annually per commuter. With 10,000 commuters, that is a $40,000,000 benefit per year, to be compared with the cost of the improvements. An intangible (leisure time) has become a dollar figure.

(Analogous price comparisons can be made in other areas than time. For instance, the appraised value of your house is based on recent prices in the sale of comparable homes.)

WILLINGNESS TO PAY

Willingness to pay (WTP) techniques are used when there is no direct market price.

Negotiated Compensation

How much are you willing to pay to keep from losing an intangible? In the Florida Keys, a noisy outdoor nightclub wanted to move next to a quiet residential area. The neighbors chipped in to buy the lot themselves. This set a WTP price on peace and quiet.

From the opposite direction, the price of a negative intangible may be determined by "willingness to accept" (WTA); that is, what a person will accept to give up an intangible. A friend moved from work in a Texas oil field to a comparable job on the north slope of Alaska. His WTA price for enduring isolation, subzero cold, and cabin fever was the extra $20,000 he received in salary.

Surrogate Market

Surrogate means "a stand-in or substitute." You can infer the value of an intangible through the surrogate market. In a condominium, there is no direct price on the value of a view. However, you can compare sale prices for internally identical apartments. If those facing the ocean on the upper floors are more expensive, you infer that the difference is the price of the view. Another example: I can get a comparable-quality broiled scallop dinner at the Red Lobster for $12 or at the more intimate Colony Inn for $20. The Colony Inn's inferred ambience price is $8.

The surrogate market can determine negative impacts as well. A major airport was planned with the approach path directly over a nearby suburban development in which the houses had been selling for $120,000. After the airport was approved, the average sale price dropped to $80,000. Based on this before and after comparison, the harm caused by noise and pollution was priced at $40,000 per family.

Hypothetical Market

Where no market currently exists, a prospective WTP price is established via a *hypothetical market*, finding out what people would be willing to pay for something. "How much wood would a woodchuck chuck, if a woodchuck could chuck wood?" A state park is considering major improvements for swimming, fishing, boating, hiking, and camping hookups financed by a $5 increase in the daily fee. It does a market survey, asking potential users whether they would use the improved facilities at the new price.

INCONSTANT DOLLARS: TIME DISCOUNTS

The use of money as a common denominator requires constant interval numbers. This means that each dollar is the same for everyone all the time. As we get more sophisticated, we recognize that not every dollar is in fact constant.

If costs and payoffs occur at about the same time, both are measured in dollars of equal value. There is no need to figure time discounts. On the other hand, in long-term planning, where costs are incurred up-front in present dollars and benefits are in future dollars, planners use *time discount* formulae to adjust the future returns back into "constant dollars."

How far into the future do you project? It is theoretically desirable to project as far into the future as any benefits will continue to result from the plan. For economic development and infrastructure planning, this could be decades. It should be at least as long as it takes you to pay back what you borrow to carry out the plan, say four years for a vehicle loan, twenty years for a mortgage, thirty years for a municipal bond.

You face a dilemma. On the one hand, if you shorten the period over which you project returns, you understate them by excluding the additional benefits of subsequent years. On the other hand, the farther into the future you project them, the less reliable become your estimates. As a planner, you have to steer between the tentacles of Scylla and the maelstrom of Charybdis, neither of which can be evaded without risking the other.

Inflation

The best known time discount is the cost-of-living index, which reduces inflated later dollars back to the $1.00 of purchasing power of a base year. If inflation goes up 25 percent, it then takes $1.25 to buy what $1.00 would buy in the base-year. To convert its value (purchasing power) to what a base-year dollar could buy, divide it by that figure. ($1.00 ÷ $1.25 = $0.80 of base-dollar purchasing power.) You can be precise in retrospect. For future projections you have to rely on the best available guesstimate of experts and trust that it will not be too far off.

Opportunity Cost

In business, the time discount is based on *opportunity cost:* what you would have earned through an alternative safe investment such as a treasury bond. This approach combines inflation and profit. For example, a 7 percent interest rate may be based on 4 percent to offset expected inflation, plus 3 percent for profit.

The process is simple arithmetic. To compare later returns with the up-front cost, compound the opportunity cost interest (7 percent in this case) annually, as follows:

```
Year  1   1.00
Year  2   1.070  (107 percent of 1.00)
Year  3   1.145  (107 percent of 1.070)
Year  4   1.225  (107 percent of 1.145)
Year  5   1.311  (107 percent of 1.225)
Year 10   1.838
```

Just as with inflation, convert each future year's return back to constant first-year dollars by dividing it by that year's adjusted opportunity cost: 1.07 the second year, 1.31 the fifth, 1.84 the tenth. Thus, the base dollar equivalent of a $1,000 payoff in the second year is $935, $763 in the fifth, and $543 in the tenth.

Deferred Gratification

"A bird in the hand is worth two in the bush." This is a deferred gratification discount, alias *"social rate of time preference."*

A young couple shared a goal of owning a home of their own. He wanted to wait until they could buy the kind of house they both wanted. This would take about five years of saving. His time preference discount was 0 percent. With a baby on the way, and unhappy with her present cramped apartment, she preferred to buy a lesser house immediately. For her, a $50,000 house now was as desirable as an $80,000 house five years from now, a time preference discount of 37.5 percent.

Retirement income, which is given full value by a person of 60, may be deeply discounted by young adults who are forty years away from the benefit. They often cash out their pension equity when changing jobs rather than rolling it over into a new account.

In economic utility theory, each person sets his or her own gratification discount rates, for whatever serious or frivolous reason. Planners don't like this, for there is no standard consistency on which to do quantitative analysis. As a compromise, some planners estimate average discounts for a population group and process the numbers as if they were hard data. How useful this is varies with the source and accuracy of its estimates.

A rate of time preference (deferral discount) of 10 percent would yield the following relative valuation of what you would accept now in lieu of the deferred benefit:

Received year 1: 1.00
Received year 2: .90
Received year 3: .81
Received year 4: .73
Received year 5: .66
Received year 10: .39

DECLINING MARGINAL UTILITY

The real price of everything, what everything really costs to the man who wants to acquire it, is the toil and trouble of acquiring it.

—Adam Smith

Marginal Utility

"You can't take it with you." Money has no value in itself, only in what it can buy. Its real value is how much "happiness" it buys you. To deal with this, we have developed the concept of *marginal utility.*

A margin is "a border." Marginal utility is "the rate of exchange [on the border] between any two competing interests, preferences, or choice." It may be the tradeoff between job and family, between watching the sunrise and sleeping in, between reading and hiking on a Saturday, between immediate profits and capital development. How much are you willing to give up from one to get (or increase) the other?

There is an *indifference point,* at which the gains and losses so exactly offset each other that the decision maker is indifferent to which way the choice goes. "Six of one or half a dozen of the other." In the economic planning model, of course, the "cost" is a dollar price, and the gain is a particular good or service, as compared with all other things you could spend the same money for. At a price below the indifference point, you will buy. At a price above that point, you will keep your money to spend on something else.

Through a complicated geometric formula, economists have devised a way to chart the average indifferent points of a population in relation to a specific commodity and dollar price (which represents everything else you could spend your money on instead). This is known as a *demand curve,* which moves across the chart from a point of low price/high demand to high price/low demand, reflecting the fact that by pushing additional buyers beyond their indifference point, each increase in price will reduce the number of buyers. This formula is not without its critics. An early skeptic warned,

> In economic theory, the assumption of mathematical continuity is very convenient. Most of geometric reasoning, based on varying types of curves, such as the demand curve, uses such an assumption. However, continuity is a deep notion and opens up the possibility of bizarre and unrealistic situations. (Little, 1957, p. 280)

The Law of Diminishing Returns

"The conventional cost benefit analysis carries an implicit weighting system; namely that one dollar is equal to one 'utile' irrespective of who gains or loses the dollar, or that a dollar gained or lost has the same value for both poor and rich," says Edward Mishan (1976, p. 404).

"It ain't necessarily so." As a teenager I had a great appetite. I could eat a whole pie at a sitting. Let's look at the value of the six pieces. On a scale of 1 to 10, the first was a 10. It took the first edge of appetite off, but the second piece was still almost as good: a 9. I was pretty satisfied before I ate the third piece, but it was still very pleasurable: call it a 7. By the fourth I was full but "there is always room for one more": a 5. The fifth piece gave little pleasure: a 2. I could still eat the sixth piece, but I didn't really want it: a 0.

This is what John Sillince (1986, p. 123) calls "the *declining marginal utility* (italics supplied) of output to the individual." The more you have, the less the next increment is worth to you. While the nominal dollars of each increment are the same, they buy less pleasure. Therefore the higher dollars are diminished.

An astute observer defined a satisfactory income as "ten percent more than whatever you have." (I think the same sage defined middle age as "ten years older than whatever you are.") If this were literally true, and the satisfaction value (marginal utility, or "U") of the next dollar increment for someone with $10,000 income is a full $1.00, the relative satisfaction value of the next dollar at different income levels would be:

$10,000	$1,000 to satisfy.	U = $1.00.
$25,000	$2,500 to satisfy.	U = $0.40.
$50,000	$5,000 to satisfy.	U = $0.20.
$100,000	$10,000 to satisfy.	U = $0.10.
$1,000,000	$100,000 to satisfy.	U = $0.01.
$30,000,000	$300,000 to satisfy.	U = 1/30 of a cent.

When basketball superstar Michael Jordan was exposed as having lost over a million dollars gambling in one year, he shrugged it off as "recreational expenditure," analogous to a fan buying a ticket to see him play. A million dollars? Ridiculous! Then I figured it in relation to diminishing marginal utility. It came out just over 3 percent of his reported income of $30,000,000. His rationale was plausible: I spent 3 percent of my salary on recreation too (and probably got as much personal pleasure from it!).

Overtime pay reflects the concept of diminishing returns in the opposite direction. Workers in a shop are willing to sell forty of their leisure hours per week, @ $10 per hour. However, with Monday through Friday filled, the remaining leisure hours for family and recreation become more valuable. It is not worth $10 per hour to give up Saturday, so the employer must pay time-and-a-half, $15, to get somebody. If the person has then worked six days, the sole remaining day of leisure becomes still more valuable, so the employer must offer double time, $20, to get a taker on Sunday. The value of another dollar relative to leisure has diminished.

When to Use Declining Marginal Utility

This is just what the doctor ordered as a partial corrective to welfare economics' indifference to distribution and the effect on individuals. With nondiminished dollars, a $1,000,000 gain for one multimillionaire is worth up to $1,000,000 worth of harm to a thousand middle-income bystanders. If its marginal utility to him is only one-tenth of what it means to them, welfare economics supports it only if the harm to them is less than $100,000. The philosophy remains unchanged, but the arithmetic leads to a less regressive distribution.

Generally, this approach is desirable:

- Where significant choices must be made among competing alternative goals.
- Where there is a significant redistribution element, with costs falling in one place and benefits another.
- Anywhere welfare economics is the planning model.

It is of less importance in relation to relatively universalistic or egalitarian benefits, such as public education or a water system, and plans which already have a progressive redistribution objective, such as low-income housing. (However, it may still be important on the financing side of the plan.)

As with so many good planning techniques and approaches, if you can't do it "by the book," you can still apply the principle informally in great and small plans. Just a common sense scan of diminishing returns may help to clarify your priorities. After such a scan, a couple who were considering a Porsche to replace their Oldsmobile decided that since they already had a fully satisfactory car, upgrading, even to a Porsche, offered less satisfaction than using those dollars to buy tuition for a midlife master's degree.

UNCERTAINTY DISCOUNT

Another major pricing factor is the *uncertainty discount*. In choosing between alternative courses of action, the price of each is arrived at through one or more of the other means we have discussed. In setting the "estimated monetary value" of each course, that price is reduced by the odds of not succeeding. (This will be discussed in Chapter 19.)

PITFALLS

It is hard to imagine making a planning choice without some kind of price comparison. However, there are a number of pitfalls to watch for. We meet some old friends here. One is faulty assumptions. The whole concept of market price as a measure or fair value is premised on the existence of a *free* market. To the extent that monopolies, regulation, fraud, and special interest lobbies subvert that "free" market, price becomes unreliable as an "objective" measure of value.

Another is "arbitrary" valuation. Once we get beyond actual market prices, the subjective judgment factor increases, reflecting the planners' values, interests, and biases. Carried to its extreme, it can be deliberately slanted: "figures don't lie but liars figure."

A third perennial problem is pseudoprecision. Sophisticated mathematical models cannot overcome inadequacies of the data, nor can aggregate patterns and curves truly represent the diverse realities in which individuals actually live.

Perhaps the greatest pitfall is the potential effect that overreliance on economic pricing can have on the intangible qualities of life, which some of us believe are the most important of all.

> To press non-economic values into the framework of the economic calculus, economists use . . . a procedure by which the

higher is reduced to the level of the lower and the priceless is given a price. . . . All it can do is lead to self-deception or the deception of others, for to undertake to measure the immeasurable is absurd and constitutes but an elaborate method of moving from preconceived notions to foregone conclusions. . . . What is worse, and destructive of civilization, is the pretense that everything has a price, or in other words, money is the highest of all values. (Schumacher, 1973, pp. 42-43)

USING PRICING METHODS

Man does live by bread—but not by bread alone. We end up with our usual multiple-method counsel: use pricing extensively in its place, but keep it there.

This array of sophisticated and helpful techniques raises a question which perhaps should be asked before we start analyzing and comparing prices. How comprehensive should it be? The answer is, enough to make a good decision in *this* plan. For some purposes, you need extensive data collection and analysis, plus such adjustments as inflation deflators and uncertainty discounts. In other situations, a rough and ready application of a few general approaches will do the job.

REFERENCES

Hayek, F. von. (1960). *The constitution of liberty.* London: Routledge & Kegan.

Keller, W. (1984). "What is the audited value of life?" *The New York Times,* October 26.

Little, I. (1957). *A critique of welfare economics.* Oxford: Oxford Press.

Merkhofer, M. (1987). *Decision science and social risk management.* Boston: D. Reidel.

Mishan, E. (1976). *Cost-benefit analysis.* 2nd ed. New York: Praeger.

Schumacher, E. (1973). *Small is beautiful.* London: Blond.

Sillince, J. (1986). *A theory of planning.* Brookfield, VT: Gower.

Chapter 18

Cost and Benefit Analyses

Thus have you heard our cause and know our means.
Then must we rate the cost of the erection,
Which if we find outweighs ability,
What do we do but draw again the model.

–Shakespeare
King Henry IV, Part II

The most widely used methods of quantitative planning analysis are based on the simple input-output economic production model presented in Chapter 4. Input is what it costs to do it; output is its result.

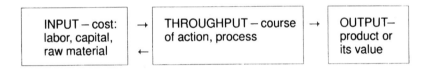

Units of value are used to measure input and output. An output unit may be each item produced, an indicator for an intangible gain, or a dollar equivalent. The output is variously called an effect, a benefit, or a utility. Commonly, all costs are measured in dollars. With these, we can compare results with what it costs to achieve them. There are three related approaches:

- *Cost effectiveness* measures input cost per unit of intended output.
- *Cost utility* measures input cost per unit of general desirability.
- *Cost benefit* measures input cost per unit of economic utility (dollars).

EFFECT: INTENDED RESULTS

An *effect* is "that which is produced by some agency or cause; a result; a consequence." In planning, "effect" is narrowed to an *intended* result (objective). We measure it by defining a unit of effect, directly or through an indicator. Since it relates only to the specified objective, it can't be compared with possible alternative uses of the same resources.

For statistical analysis and comparisons, the measures of effect must be in constant interval numbers. At the simplest level, this can be a yes (1) or no (0) category. In an adoption program, a completed adoption is a "1." A more sophisticated interval scale can differentiate the degree of success. For an electric power plant, it may be a kilowatt hour produced. In a remedial reading program for second graders, may be a point gained on a standardized before-and-after reading test.

BENEFIT: RESULTS IN DOLLARS

The generic definition of benefit is "anything that is for the good of a person or thing." Conventional planning narrows it to the *money value* of the good thing. Although it can be applied to an individual's outcomes, it is most widely used to calculate overall payoff for large systems, such as a corporation, a community, or the entire economy.

Its big advantage over effectiveness is that its common denominator of value lets you compare the relative desirability of different choices. It suffers the limitations discussed in the chapters on economics and pricing.

UTILITY: NONMONETARY GOODNESS MEASURES

"Utility" is used to refer to any nonmonetary common denominator of goodness on which the planners can agree. I call utility units "goody points." Utility can also measure "baddy points" (diswelfares). Subtracting them from the goody points yields a net goodness score.

Utility might be used in determining priority for rationed organ transplants, where only one-third of those with the need can be served. You have rejected the traditional economic standard of valuing a life solely on future earning potential, yet you must still decide whose life is saved and who will be left to die. You can, of course, reject any consideration of utility by using a random chance lottery, but is that the best use of your limited resources? One medical team used a year of additional healthy life as the unit. Thus, those with better general health prognoses get more points than those who would still be severely disabled, and a 40-year-old candidate gets more points than an equally healthy 70-year-old.

Utility is used less often than effectiveness or benefit for two reasons. One is that it is more difficult to quantify precisely. The other is getting voluntary agreement on the utility point criteria. The transplant utility illustration above may be vulnerable to both these problems.

The size of the project makes a difference. In personal and small homogeneous group planning, this may not be an issue. On the other hand, in large-scale planning where diverse parties have different values and preferences, it is almost impossible to achieve consensus.

A common utility technique is a rating scale, such as 1 to 10, or the simple, popular +2 to -2 scale: very good (2), good (1), neutral (0), bad (-1), very bad (-2). Each result gets a score. This is often a subjective value judgment. Such judgments are acceptable for planning if they (1) are made in a conscious, consistent way, and (2) represent the consensus decision makers. It becomes less reliable, however, if the valuations are being made by more than one person, due to normal human differences in interpretation and judgments, as in the case of GPA, with its diversity of professor-graders.

The utility approach can also be used to determine the relative value (weight) of different effects. One approach uses 1.00 as ideal, and weighs other alternatives against it. For instance, in a permanence for children program, there are six possible outcomes. Let us say the following utility weighting was applied:

- Restoration of the child's home of origin   1.00
- Permanent adoption by a relative, 80% as desirable   .80

- Adoption by a nonrelative .70
- Long-term foster care without the security of adoption .50
- Long-term institutionalization .30
- No permanent arrangement, shunted around .10
- Abandonment .00

The needs exceed the resources of the agency. There are now four children in foster care ($4 \times .50 = 2.00$) and one in an institution ($.30$) for a utility score of 2.30. There is enough money in next year's budget to pay for either (A) the restoration of one family which had neglected or abused the child, or (B) five adoptions. The utility score of (A) is one restoration ($= 1.00$), plus three left in foster care ($3 \times .50 = 1.50$), and one in an institution ($= .30$): a total of 2.80 utility points. The score of all five adopted is 3.50 ($5 \times .70$). Therefore, five adoptions are a better use of the resources than one restoration. (If the utility weighting of desirability were changed, the answer would come out different.)

Another common weighting system starts at a minimal standard, 1.0, and gives higher weights to more valuable effects. In some universities, utility of a student credit hour (SCH) is valued differently at each level in calculating a professor's "productivity":

- Lower division (freshman-sophomore) 1.0
- Upper division (junior-senior) 1.5
- Master's 2.0
- Doctoral 3.0

With this weighting, a professor's "production" is valued the same (36 utility points) for a class with 12 doctoral students, 18 Master's students, 24 seniors, or 36 freshmen.

SIDE EFFECTS

We now return to the broader definition of "effect" as "*any* result of an action." The objectives of the plan are intended effects, the ones measured for cost effectiveness. There are also other results, not intended. These are *side effects*, alias:

- *Byproducts:* "something produced in the process of making another thing: secondary or incidental product or result."
- *Spillover* effects: "not deliberately produced and not deliberately absorbed by others" (Mishan, 1976, p. 111).
- *Ripple* effects: a pattern of side effects which go out and out, spreading farther afield in a more complex pattern than a mere nearside spill.
- *Externalities:* all effects which fall outside the defined boundaries of the plan.
- *Counterintuitive consequences:* unexpected side effects.
- *Epiphenomena* (for lovers of obscure but accurate words): "facts or circumstances that occur with and seem to result from another."

Characteristics

Side effects may be economic, social, physical, psychological, or aesthetic. Utility techniques are flexible enough to incorporate side effects. Cost effectiveness, by definition, excludes them. Benefit analysis can encompass any side effect which can be priced in dollars. However, it rarely makes the effort: "Usually such costs and benefits are those accruing directly to the decision-maker, so that 'externalities' are ignored" (Sillince, 1986, p. 123).

Side effects can be positive, a bonus. For instance, the objective of Social Security is individual income security in old age or disability. A side effect of this is to lessen the extremes of economic cycles because 15 percent of the population maintains a stable, "recession proof" demand.

Some side effects may be more valuable than the original intent. A wise, opportunistic planner will be alert for *serendipity*, "the faculty of making desirable but unsought-for discoveries by accident." A famous case is the "Hawthorne effect." Efficiency engineers at Westinghouse developed a plan to increase production through brighter lighting. As it turned out, the lighting itself had minimal effect, but a side effect was that workers' morale increased in response to the company's taking an interest in them. *This* raised production. Learning from this, a new human relations approach to administrative planning was developed.

Side effects can be negative. A classic illustration is the

"Monkey's Paw" tale. A couple were given a monkey's paw that would grant three wishes. They wished for a large sum of money. They got it. There was a side effect: it was insurance from their only child's death in a gory accident. So they wished the son back to life. The side effect: excruciating pain from the injury. They used the third wish to relieve him of his pain—which was achieved, you guessed it, by his dying again.

Some side effects are anticipated, some unexpected, and some unrecognized. To illustrate, let's look at some of the effects of the Medicare/Medicaid programs established in 1965:

- *Intended effect:* adequate health care for the aged and poor.
- *Anticipated side effect:* enrich doctors, hospitals, and pharmaceuticals. Indeed, this side effect was exchanged for withdrawal of opposition.
- *Unexpected effects.* Conventional expectations were that payment for many former charity cases would "save" the hard-pressed nonprofit hospital sector. However, the actual effect was to commercialize the field. Whereas business had avoided a sure money loser, public (and expanding private) insurance third-party payments converted it into a potential money maker. (In retrospect, we should have anticipated this as a normal side effect in a market economy.)
- *Unrecognized effects.* We rarely note iatrogenic ("caused by medical treatment") disorders as a side effect.

Generally speaking, it is best to anticipate as many side effects as possible. This enables us to make the best planning choice and to encounter fewer unpleasant surprises.

We should be particularly alert for unrecognized effects, for we can do great harm in our ignorance. For instance, unaware of an iatrogenic factor, our planning response to an increase in certain health problems might be to exacerbate the problem by adding still more iatrogenic services.

Including and Ignoring Side Effects

An ethical fairness principle says that all stakeholders affected by the outcome should be taken into account. This calls for attention to side effects in general. More specifically, such attention may be called for in the following situations:

- You have reason to expect significant side effects.
- The actions will have predictable negative effects on bystanders. When we spray a mosquito infested area, the crickets are silenced and the population of swallows and martins is decimated. Is it still a net gain?
- The plan involves redistribution. You need to know from whom, to whom, how much?
- You are committed to compensatory Pareto Improvement and aware that, as the world turns, most of the "losers" will be bystanders damaged by side effects.
- Positive side effects can help sell your plan, such as Medicare's side effect of raising physicians' income, and food stamps' side effect of increasing demand and prices for farmers' products.

On the other hand, in modest, compartmental planning, the spillover impact is minimal, not worth getting into. If I buy a house, it theoretically affects the whole economy through the "invisible hand" of free market process. So does a drop of rain affect the ocean. But not enough for me to bother about.

In general, you can give low priority to side effects that neither hurt others nor affect a plan's support and acceptance.

Side effects may be ignored for an entirely different reason. Self-centered planning is focused only on the "main chance," indifferent to its wider impacts. Many consider this to be ethical in socially-sanctioned competitive situations. When you win a career promotion, you are not lying awake nights worrying about the disappointment of a coworker. Corporations do not worry about how their actions affect their competitors' profits.

Even in the above circumstances, there can still be strategic benefits from knowing how the side effects fall. At the very least, we should do a quick scan.

INPUT: COST

The dictionary gives two definitions of "cost" which apply to cost and benefit analyses. The first is "the amount spent in producing or manufacturing a commodity." The second is "loss, sacrifice, detriment," which includes all negative effects, wherever they may fall.

For a small-scale personal plan, such as a semester course load, the cost might be in terms of two inputs: approximate time required and an experience-based estimate of stress. As the inputs increase in number and complexity, however, they become harder to handle intuitively. A do-it-the-hard-way older student may need to factor in the costs of tuition, lost earnings, daycare, and intangible side effects on loved ones.

PROGRAM BUDGETING

In any complex plan, the factors will be multiple, and you can calculate and compare overall costs only if you convert all specific costs to a numerical common denominator. Nearly all formal planning uses money, assessed through standard budgeting and accounting methods.

The old "line item" cash budget system used an agency-wide line for each "object category" (rent, equipment, salaries, benefits, postage, etc.) containing the dollars actually spent (or to be spent) in each. This was fine until the advent of cost effectiveness and cost-benefit analyses. Under the old system, there was no way to know what part of the agency budget was spent on any particular product, nor how much "in kind" (noncash) input cost there was.

The solution: *program budgeting*. Each agency function is separately identified, with a vertical column in which all of its direct costs are enumerated. The object category lines are retained but broken down by function. For instance, "salaries" are allocated among columns for basic classroom learning, special education, music, sports, administration, etc. Each column adds its line items to a total direct cost of performing the function.

Functions fall into two categories: *direct programs* and *indirect support*. Each direct program has *one* measurable specific objective (product). In our permanence for children agency, those programs may be protection (investigation of alleged abuse and neglect), family restoration (therapy, parenting education), foster home care, institutional care, and adoption.

The second type of function is *indirect* general support, popularly called "overhead." In the charitable sector this consists of two functions: management-and-general and fundraising. Into the latter go all management other than direct supervision of specific programs: the CEO's office, accounting, personnel office, and community relations. It is also the catchall for shared support services which cannot be precisely allocated, such as a waiting room and receptionist.

The preliminary steps are:

- Identify each separate specific objective as a program.
- Set up a separate budget for each program.
- For each program identify every ingredient for pricing.
- Do the same for each general support function.

Next, calculate direct program costs. Put in all items which are fully devoted to the objective: worker and direct supervisor salaries and benefits, staff travel expenses, toll calls, and departmental supplies and equipment. If you use a separate administrative unit for each program, you are off and running because you can blanket in its entire budget with no further ado.

For example, if a staff person divides her time among more than one program, her FTE (full time equivalence) must be allocated proportionately among the programs. If she works three days per week in Oncology and two days in Dialysis, her total FTE costs should be divided as 60 percent (.60) and 40 percent (.40). Theoretically, this should be based on a daily time log. It is cheaper and almost as accurate to use periodic sampling methods. It is still cheaper, and close enough for most purposes, to use an official administrative time allocation—provided it honestly reflects the actual time spent.

There are simple standard methods for allocating the program's share of other costs. For instance, instead of calculating separate rent, utilities, and maintenance for each office, get agency-wide line-budget costs and allocate as each program's share the percentage of floor space its offices occupy. If a program uses 500 of the agency's 5,000 sq. ft., allocate 10 percent of all agency occupancy costs to it. Similar methods can be based on percentage usage of the Xerox machine, percent of telephone extensions, etc.

You should identify any costs hidden in another program budget. For instance, by informal mutual agreement, a psychology professor teaches a social work course once per year. Strict program budgeting requires that the 10 percent (.10) of his FTE used to teach the course should show as a social work education rather than psychology program cost. (In this actual case, they decided it didn't make enough difference to bother about: not kosher, but perhaps a common sense application of the Law of Parsimony.)

All nonmoney costs are converted to their dollar equivalent. Staff time becomes salary and benefits. A volunteer hour becomes the "would have been" staff-time cost. A donated secondhand word processor becomes $200. This is relatively easy.

The most serious flaw in the conversion-to-dollars system is a familiar one, the tendency to ignore or undervalue hard-to-measure intangible costs, such as the "hidden" costs of poorer quality and increased error rate caused by overloads assigned as an alleged cost-cutting measure. Perhaps we can offset such limitations by bringing overlooked elements into the full decision-making mix in some other way.

Now that we have all the direct program costs, we add up all the support function costs, using the same system, then dump into it whatever is left that we can't reliably allocate directly.

To get *total program cost*, divide the support function costs equitably among the programs. The conventional criterion for allocation of general support is size of budget. If one program is 25 percent of the aggregate direct program budgets, 25 percent of the overhead is tacked onto it.

This works pretty well most of the time, but sometimes one should be a little more careful. For instance, fundraising support costs should be allocated only among programs supported by those funds, with none charged off to a program that is self-supporting through fees. Another variable is how much support is actually received by the program. A routine high-budget program may need only half as much management and support as an experimental pilot program with one-tenth as much budget.

The cost of any plan is all inputs, including those that failed to produce, while at the output end only successful effects are counted.

For instance, a family counseling agency treats 100 cases at a cost of $500 each ($50,000). Only half are successful. The total cost, however, is still $50,000. (This makes the agency cost per successful case $50,000 ÷ 50, or $1,000.)

COST EFFECTIVENESS

Cost effectiveness (CE) is the same as *efficiency*, "ability to produce the desired effect with a minimum of effort, expense, or waste." It is the most modest of the three cost-result comparisons. It does not ask whether an objective is worth doing or how it compares with other objectives. What it *does* do well is to compare alternative means to achieve the same predetermined objective.

Fixed Utility versus Fixed Budget

While the basic arithmetic is the same, CE can be approached from opposite perspectives and intents. *Fixed utility* seeks to accomplish the *same* effect more cheaply. For example, there is reason to believe that for some patients, group therapy is as effective as individual sessions, which cost twice as much per person. By shifting to more group and less individual sessions, we expect to achieve the same success for less cost.

In the *fixed budget* approach, the aim is to "get more bang for the buck," as the Pentagon used to say. This is especially appropriate where available resources are externally set (by appropriation, budget allocation, personal income, or economic cycles). Make the most of whatever you have.

Using the same data, let's see how the two approaches are applied. An adoption program has had 32 successful placements with a budget of $160,000 ($5,000 each). It then becomes more cost effective, lowering the unit cost to $4,000. A fixed utility CE application would maintain the 32 placements next year with a reduced budget of $128,000. The same agency, with a fixed-budget approach, would shoot for 40 placements next year with the same $160,000 budget that placed 32 last year.

Both approaches can be used in the same plan. One may use fixed utility in relation to a specific objective within a plan that is using a fixed-budget approach at the strategic level. Money saved by using more group therapy to serve the same number of adults may be used to expand the therapeutic pre-school program.

Total versus Marginal Comparisons

There are two ways to apply cost effectiveness. One is to compare the *total* revised cost with the total revised effect. The other is to compare only the incremental changes on the *margin*; that is, compare the new costs with the new effects.

An open admissions public college spends $1,000,000 on 100 new freshmen. Half of them flunk out. The CE of the 50 successes is $20,000 each. If you spend $1,000 each to tutor the 50 poor students ($50,000) and get 20 more successes, the marginal cost is $2,500 per success in the new program. If instead you spend $2,000 for a combined tutoring and counseling service and 30 of them succeed, its marginal cost is $3,333. Which program is more cost effective? It depends on how you look at it. Marginally, tutor-only is. However from the total program perspective, which includes the basic $10,000 spent per student, the tutor-counseling is more cost effective.

	Marginal			Total		
	Cost	Effect	CE	Cost	Effect	CE
No change	$0	0	$0	$1,000,000	50	$20,000
Tutor only	$50,000	20	$2,500	$1,050,000	70	$15,000
Tutor-counsel	$100,000	30	$3,333	$1,100,000	80	$13,750

Where It Goes Wrong

The greatest pitfall of cost effectiveness is not in its methodology but how often it is misapplied. Spurious cost effectiveness is an "under the streetlight" error which substitutes units of *input* for units of *outcome*. This can subvert goal-oriented planning in several ways:

- Goal displacement from results to activities: bureaucratic thinking.
- Simple cost containment, where the aim is to cut expenses without reference to the effects. Low success rates in several

large public social programs result from their hiring cheaper, unqualified workers to carry oversize caseloads (reducing the cost per case) with few successes, rather than professionals who would cost more and carry fewer cases, but move clients successfully off the rolls.

• Complacency, created by the de facto implication that if we are judged by inputs, then input is tantamount to success. It squelches proper attention to evaluating and improving real effectiveness.

This is especially tempting in human services where we have difficulty trying to measure nonmaterial effects. A charitable federation required program budgeting of its agencies as part of a cost effectiveness review. However, instead of asking its agencies for a report on hard-to-measure units of effect (client outcomes), it had them report easy-to-count units of input to the clients (contact hours or number of persons served).

Such displacement has escalated health care costs. Insurance has traditionally measured (and rewarded) inputs only (physician, operating room, anesthesia, bed care, meals, medicines, etc.) without reference to what happened–good, bad, or indifferent–to the patient. This encourages providers to order unnecessary (but profitable) procedures.

Medicare countered this with a flat rate for each of several hundred Diagnostically Related Groups (DRGs) of disorders, regardless of itemized inputs. It succeeded in discouraging unnecessary costs, but because it still ignored effect, it substituted a new displacement: an incentive to cut corners on care regardless of how it affected the patient.

COST-BENEFIT ANALYSIS

The House of Representatives Tuesday approved far-reaching changes in how federal agencies enforce health, safety, and environmental laws. It directed regulatory agencies to base rules primarily on economic calculations of costs and benefits. Statistics and finances would override the health-based standards at the heart of many existing environmental laws. . . .

Decisions about everything from automobile safety standards and workplace rules to emissions from smokestacks and the purification of drinking water could be changed.

—The New York Times, March 1, 1995

Cost-benefit analysis is a businesslike way of making choices. There are two basic concepts. One is *profit*. Will the results be worth more than the cost of doing something? "Cost benefit analysis is a procedure for 1) measuring the gains and losses to individuals, using money as the measuring rod of those gains and losses, and 2) aggregating the many valuations of the gains and losses of the individuals and expressing them as net social gains and losses" (Pearce, 1983, p. 3).

A related concept is *opportunity* cost. To achieve any objective, we must use resources (cash, materials, facilities, personnel, time, etc.) which we convert to dollar costs. In our finite world, if we use them to achieve opportunity A, they are not available for opportunity B or C. If we use them for C, we can't do A or B. You have enough money to make a down payment on a house, invest in the stock market, or pay for advance training which will upgrade your future earnings–but only for one of them. Which should you pick? You have met the opportunity cost test if your choice offers a better payoff than any other.

Using Cost Benefit Analysis

Cost benefit analysis (CBA) has a long history. The formal analytical technique was developed by Jules Dupuit, a French economist and engineer, and published in 1844 in his *On Measuring of Utility of Public Works*.

It became a mainstream planning "model" through a version called Program Planning Budgeting System (PPBS). The approach was developed by the Army Corps of Engineers in the 1920s, adopted by some corporations, and brought to Washington by a former corporation CEO, Robert McNamara. It spread from the Pentagon to domestic programs and human services, and through government grant and contract requirements to the private sectors. Although the next administration dismantled it, the approach remains widely used (at least in lip service) by corporations, public agencies, and the nonprofit sector, which revised its entire set of audit standards to fit it.

The key elements of *CBA* are:

- Product-based cost accounting: what a product *really* costs.
- Dollar pricing of that product.
- A comparison of costs and benefits to determine which course of action offers the best deal.

The appeal of cost-benefit analysis is that all costs and benefits are valued in dollars. Because everyone uses this common denominator every day, it is easily understood. Because everything is reduced to one measure, virtually anything can be compared with anything else. Because the results are neat, clean, and statistical, they carry an aura of credibility and offer escape from ambiguity. Because it deals in economic bottom lines, it is a (literally) businesslike approach.

CBA can show whether something is worth doing. Add up the benefit dollars, subtract the cost dollars and *voila!—the bottom line.* If it is a gain, the plan is worth doing.

If, on the other hand, it shows a net loss by costing more than the result is worth, beware. It might lead to a *pyrrhic victory.* In 279 B.C., King Pyrrhus of Epirus invaded Italy and dealt the Romans a resounding defeat at Asculum. However, his casualties were high and his replacement/supply lines were overextended. Several months later, the Romans, with new citizen soldiers to replace their slaughtered army, fought him again in his depleted condition. He was chased out of Italy, and before long lost his throne back home in Epirus.

CBA can do more than tell you *whether.* It can tell you *how* profitable. This is particularly helpful in selecting the best among several good choices. It uses a simple formula: $B/C = R$ (ratio of benefit-to-cost). If you estimate a $110 benefit from a $100 cost, your $110/$100 ratio equals 1.1. This qualifies as worth doing, but not as good as B, with a $200 benefit for the $100 cost, B/C ratio of 2.0, a doubling of the investment.

CBA presumes that unless proven otherwise, the best course of action is the one with the highest B/C ratio. If you are a purist it *dictates* the choice. "The basic premise of cost benefit theory is that alternatives should be selected according to a systematic comparison of the advantages and disadvantages that result from the estimated consequences of choice" (Merkhofer, 1987, p. 60).

There are other considerations, such as ethics, equity of distribution of gains and losses, political tradeoffs, and personal interest. The most profitable aggregate course may also be the most damaging to vulnerable bystanders. It may make you unpopular with voters and powerful lobbyists. You may simply find the less profitable venture more interesting and fun. Even so, you will probably try to get as close to the optimum benefit/cost ratio as the other factors permit.

CBA is waived when the result is so important that it transcends any consideration of cost, as in the crisis mobilization of munitions manufacture in World War II. The government resorted to "cost-plus." Spend whatever it takes and we will pay that cost plus a reasonable profit on top. It was a calculated decision that worked when it had to. However, such disregard of CBA in noncrisis circumstances is seen as fiscally irresponsible and/or corrupt.

Limitations

The clear advantages of CBA are qualified by the limitations we have already identified in pseudoscience, quantification, economic reductionism, and defects of pricing indicators. Much of this stems from a quest for neat and clean statistics at the expense of harder-to-measure intangible costs and benefits. Its ideological ties to welfare economics' impersonal dismissal of individual interests and effects are controversial.

No one who works with cost-benefit analysis should fail to read Jonathan Swift's devastating 1729 satire on CBA (before it was officially invented): *A Modest Proposal for Preventing the Children of the Poor People of Ireland from Being a Burden to Their Parents or Country, and for Making them Beneficial to the Public.*

In Its Place

Cost benefit analysis as traditionally practiced is no more than a useful technique in the service of social decisions. . . . The

outcome of a cost-benefit analysis alone is not socially deci-
sive. A cost benefit analysis neglects distributional effects. It
neglects equity. It may have to ignore spillover effects. . . . In
summary, a cost benefit study can be *only a part, though an
important part* (italics supplied) of the data necessary for informed collective decisions. (Mishan, 1976, pp. 412-13)

Use it with two qualifications. First of all, use CBA as one of
multiple inputs to the decision. Alone, "we see mean-minded and
heartless bureaucrats thinking like computers" (Merkhofer, 1987,
p. 177). Blended with the qualitative and experiential perspectives
of nonscientific rationality, it helps produce a "combination of a
cool head and a warm heart . . . [shielded from] sentimentality on
the one hand and indifference on the other" (Howard, 1980).

Second, use it as a servant, not a master. Identify your VIBES
explicitly. Know what they are. Be sure that the CBA pricing reflects those VIBES. Make this overt so that other decision makers
can take it into account.

COST UTILITY

Cost utility is cost per unit of human satisfaction, however measured.

People usually choose either cost effectiveness (CE) or cost-
benefit analysis (CBA). CE is an efficient tool where there is commitment to the objective (ends), so that the only issue is which way
to do it (means). CBA helps to choose a course of action which
includes both ends and means.

Cost utility is a flexible compromise to fall back on when neither
of the other two quite fit. It uses a common measure of value for all
effects, so that, like CBA, it can compare the merits of diverse
objectives. Unlike CBA, it is not shackled to economic reductionism. For example, my program has an elective course which reportedly requires greater cost in time, work, and anxiety than any other
which offers the same credit, yet it is also our most popular elective.
Why? Because it tops our students' (implicit) "learning value"
utility scale. (With a smile, I promote it to advisees on a CBA basis
too: "Hey, you get five credits worth of training for only three
credits' tuition cost!")

When is cost utility least desirable? In large complex plans, where there is considerable social, cultural, and interest diversity; in a business corporation, where the bottom line really is dollars; and in economic and financial planning projects.

Where may cost utility be most useful? In compartmental planning, where an individual, family, or small group share a high consensus on the definition of what is good.

It is also desirable in specific situations where dollars simply won't cut the mustard. Where intangibles that cannot be measured in economic terms are critically important, an imperfect cost utility review may be more valid than a wonderfully neat analysis of the wrong thing. War is inappropriate for evaluation on the basis of economic cost benefit. Lives lost and saved may be more appropriate as utility units.

REFERENCES

Howard, R. (1980). "An assessment of decision analysis." *Operations Research*, 28.

Merkhofer, M. (1987). *Decision science and social risk management*. Boston: D. Reidel.

Mishan, E. (1976). *Cost-benefit analysis*. 2nd ed. New York: Praeger.

Pearce, D. (1983). *Cost benefit analysis*. London: Macmillan.

Sillince, J. (1986). *A theory of planning*. Brookfield, VT: Gower.

Chapter 19

Playing the Odds: Decision Analysis

Nothing is more certain than incertainties;
Fortune is full of fresh variety:
Constant in nothing but inconstancy.

–Richard Barnfield, ca. 1600

ROOM FOR UNCERTAINTY

In an old fable, the animals had already filled a Christmas stocking to the brim when the little mouse's turn came. The other animals taunted that he could put nothing more in it. "Yes I can," he replied, and put a hole in the heel.

We have filled up our stocking with values and interests, key result areas, goals and means, desirability and feasibility, costs and benefits, indifference curves and shadow pricing, scientific quantification and intuition . . . and who knows what-all. It is chock full.

All information, whether systematic or experiential, shares a common characteristic: it is from the past, what has already occurred. But all plans take place in the future. There is still room for a hole, *uncertainty.* We can never be sure.

It is appropriate, then, that our final technique, *decision analysis* (DA), is an effort to darn the hole using best-guess numbers as the thread and simple arithmetic as the needle. It simplifies a complex pattern to manageable components, each of which is plotted separately and then calculated in with the others.

Uncertainty is made more severe by being compounded into a chain of events. It is hard enough to make an assessment of probabilities in the case of a single action with several outcomes but it is much more difficult to make a set of mutually consistent probability assessments for a whole chain of outcomes. . . . The manager has to solve these problems in any case. Regardless of whether or not he writes anything down, uses formulae, or has ever heard of Bayes' strategies, he is balancing uncertainty in some way. The contention of modern decision theory is that it is better to have some formal procedure for dealing with uncertainty because that at least makes the judgment explicit and open to discussion by those involved. (Coyle, 1972, p. 24)

CAUSES AND EFFECTS

The purpose of planning is to cause an effect. A *decision* among competing alternatives is based on the best available projection of probable causes and effects. Three kinds of variables come into play:

- *Dependent* variables are effects, results, outcomes, or, in DA, "events." Goals and objectives are dependent variables.
- *Independent* variables are recognized and controllable causes of an effect. Means apply independent variables.
- An *intervening* variable is an uncontrolled element which may affect the outcome. Contingencies are the result of intervening variables.

Before applying DA, use basic planning methods to reduce possible alternative objectives to serious finalists, so that you don't waste time charting, evaluating, and calculating probabilities for things you aren't going to do anyway.

To keep it (relatively) simple, don't try to factor everything in. It should be limited to key elements in five areas:

1. *Choices* within your control (*independent* variables).
2. *Contingency* factors beyond your control (*intervening* variables).
3. Possible alternative *results* of each choice due to contingencies (*dependent* variables).
4. The *probability* of each possible result actually occurring.
5. The *value* of each possible result if it occurs.

THE DECISION TREE

A popular model is the *decision tree*, a diagram that breaks complex decision problems down into a sequential structure which follows out the branching effects of both choice and contingency variables.

- A *fork* is a point at which alternatives split.
- A *choice fork* is a point where you can choose among alternative courses of action.
- A *contingency fork* is a point at which uncontrolled factors affect the outcome.
- *Branches* are alternative choices or contingencies going out from a fork.
- The outcome at the end of each branch is an *event*.
- A *chain* is a sequence of branches.
- The outcome at the end of each chain is the *terminal event*.
- *Scenario* is "an outline of the plot of a dramatic work, giving the action in the order in which it takes place and specification as to scenes, situations, and casts of characters." In DA, a scenario is the step-by-step tree layout from a starting point to the whole range of possible outcomes, including all forks, branches, chains, and events–the plot of a plan with specification as to scenes and situations.

Below is a potential social work training applicant's simple decision tree.

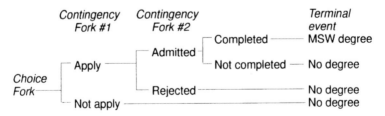

The choice fork has two branches: whether to apply or not. If you don't apply, there are no contingencies, and the terminal event is no degree. If you do apply, the first contingency point is whether you are admitted. If rejected, your terminal event is also no degree. If admitted, you move down the chain to the next contingency fork: whether you complete the program or not. The terminal event at the end of the "completed" branch is the MSW. The terminal event for the unable-to-complete branch is no degree.

PROBABILITIES

Two Kinds of Odds

Decision analysts predict the impact of uncontrolled intervening variables: the percentage probability (P) of each possible result which could occur from a given course of action.

They recognize two kinds. *Deterministic* odds are known, as in flipping coins, drawing to an inside straight, or trying a finesse in bridge. They are called *objective* probability. The conditions are known. I don't know whether heads or tails will come up in this coin flip, but I do know I have exactly a 50/50 chance of getting tails: no more, no less. Knowing the odds, I take a calculated risk.

Decision analysts are practical folk. If they don't know the actual odds, they make an educated guess, called *subjective*, or *stochastic* ("inferring, theorizing, or predicting from incomplete or uncertain evidence") probability. More often than not, this guesstimate is the best we can do. A bookie's point spread for next Saturday's football game is stochastic.

The Bayesian Approach

The classical DA approach is "Bayesian." Bayes was an Anglican priest who developed the mathematical theory of gambling.

The *Bayes Theorem* is the cornerstone of all decision analysis. It states that *the probabilities of all possible mutually exclusive outcomes of a given cause must add up to 1.00 (100 percent)*. For instance, this morning the weatherman predicts the probability of two outcomes this evening: rain or no rain. He forecasts a 60 percent probability of rain, which means the chance of no rain is 40 percent.

The estimate at the outset is called *prior* probability. As we gain experience and information along the way, we may revise the probability estimates for the remainder of the plan and make adjustments accordingly. These are called *posterior* probabilities. At noon, our weatherman, observing an intensifying front, updates the forecast to 80 percent probability of evening rain (and 20 percent no rain).

Due to uncontrolled circumstances, a specific action choice might lead to several different outcomes (events). The likelihood of any particular direct event resulting from a specific action choice is called its *simple* (or *unconditional* or *marginal*) probability. (The Ps of all possible alternative events from this action will, of course, add up to 100 percent.)

Joint Probability

Events are often linked together, with each subsequent event dependent on the prior one having occurred. This is called a Markhov chain. The probability of the down-the-line event is the *joint probability* (JP): a combination of its own (simple) P with the P of its prerequisite.

What are my chances of getting three tails in a row, if there is a 50 percent chance on each coin flip? The P of tails on the first flip is .50. The JP of two tails in a row is that .50 of one tail times its .50 chance on the second flip (.50 $\times$ .50 = .25). The JP of three in a row is that .25 chance of two in a row times the .50 of the third: .125 (12.5 percent).

English 101 is a prerequisite for 102. My P of passing 101, and therefore becoming eligible to take 102, is 80 percent. My P of passing 102 if I take it is 90 percent. My JP, therefore, of a successful completion of the two-course chain is .80 $\times$ .90, or 72 percent.

Let's see how this works for the applicant in the decision tree shown earlier.

1st Event	P	2nd Event	P	JP	Terminal Event P
		FINISH	.90	.63	.63
ADMIT	.70				
APPLY MSW		DROP	.10	.07	.07
REJECT	.30				.30
	(1.00)		(1.00)		(1.00)

Seventy percent of applicants are admitted. 90 percent of admitted students complete the program. The JP of getting in and getting out is

63 percent (.70 × .90) and of acceptance but not graduating is 7 percent (.70 × .10). The P of not getting in is 30 percent. The set of alternative terminal events adds up to 100 percent.

ESTIMATED VALUE OF EACH CHOICE

The likelihood of an event occurring is only half the battle. The other half is its payoff (or loss) if it does occur. This is called *estimated value* (EV), and is arrived at through the cost-benefit analysis method. While any numerical unit of value may be used, DA customarily uses estimated *monetary* value (EMV).

Average Estimated Value

If you mix red and white paint, the blend will be in between. How dark or light depends on the proportion of the two colors. With just a dash of red, you may get a rose-tinted off-white. With lots of red, you have a robust blushing pink.

Proportional averaging can be illustrated by a composite wage for two part-time jobs. The weekly full-time equivalent pay is $800 for job A, and $500 for B. If you work both half-time, your average pay will be $650 per week (1/2 of $800 = $400; 1/2 of $500 = $250). If instead you work 75 percent at A and only 25 percent at B, it will be $725 (3/4 of $800 = $600; 1/4 of $500 = $125).

DA uses a similar approach to estimating average EMV of all the possible outcomes of a chosen course of action, giving proportional weight to each possible outcome according to its relative probability.

The *Bayesian Formula* (based on Bayes' theorem) does this. It estimates the probability of each possible outcome of a given choice actually occurring (adding up to 100 percent of course) and the value of each should it occur. Let's say there are three possible outcomes:

> #1, which has a 60 percent probability, is worth $100 if it occurs.
> #2, which has a 25 percent probability, is worth $200 if it occurs.
> #3, which has a 15 percent probability, is worth $300 if it occurs.

To get the average estimated value of the whole mix, you add 60 percent of #1 ($60), 25 percent of #2 ($50) and 15 percent of #3 ($45), for an average value of $155, which you can compare with a similarly calculated average value of each other course of action under consideration.

Illustration

Let's see how this works in practice on a doctoral-masters decision tree. You are a "psych tech" who wants to upgrade to professional therapist. Your college GPA was in the B+ range. You have narrowed the choice of routes to either a five-year PhD in psychology or a two-year master's in Social Work. A third choice is to forget the whole thing and remain a tech. We have a scenario for each of these choices. Based on probable earnings over the next twenty years, which is your best choice?

We have earlier calculated the probabilities for the apply-MSW choice of an MSW application. Let us do the same for the apply-PhD and not-apply choices:

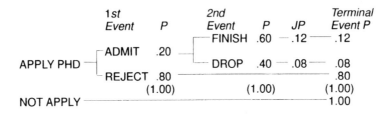

	1st Event	P	2nd Event	P	JP	Terminal Event P
			FINISH	.60	.12	.12
	ADMIT	.20				
APPLY PHD			DROP	.40	.08	.08
	REJECT	.80				.80
		(1.00)		(1.00)		(1.00)
NOT APPLY						1.00

Combined with our earlier MSW choice, we now have the probability of all possible terminal events. Next we calculate the monetary value of each terminal event: expected gains minus costs. In this case, there are three salary levels: $80,000 per year worked for the PhD, $40,000 for the MSW, and $20,000 for the tech. A year of training costs $10,000 (in addition to losing a year of earnings). We will estimate it for a twenty-year period from the date of the application decision.

- PhD. Net EV = $1,150,000: 15 working years @ $80,000 ($1,200,000) minus five years of training expenses @$10,000 ($50,000).

- MSW. Net EV = $700,000: 18 working years @ $40,000 ($720,000) minus two years of training expenses ($20,000).
- Tech. Net EV = $400,000: 20 working years @ 20,000, no training expense.
- Drop out (after a year of training). Net EV = $370,000: 19 years @ $20,000 ($380,000), minus $10,000 for one year of training expenses.

Finally we develop an average EMV for each choice by a proportional composite of the possible events of each choice.

	Terminal Event P		Event EMV		Proportional Share
PhD					
1. Apply-admit-finish	.12	×	$1,150,000	=	$138,000
2. Apply-admit-drop out	.08	×	$ 370,000	=	$ 29,600
3. Apply-reject	.80	×	$ 400,000	=	$320,000
Average EMV	*(1.00)*				*$487,600*
MSW					
1. Apply-admit-finish	.63	×	$ 700,000	=	$441,000
2. Apply-admit-drop out	.07	×	$ 370,000	=	$ 25,900
3. Apply-reject	.30	×	$ 400,000	=	$120,000
Average EMV	*(1.00)*				*$586,900*
Not Apply					
Average EMV	*1.00*		*$ 400,000*		*$400,000*

The average EMV method, does *not* tell you what the outcome value will actually be for the choice in this particular instance. (It will be one of the specific outcomes, better or worse than the composite.) It *does* give you information on which to take a calculated risk, namely what the average value of 100 cases would be (assuming your probability estimates are accurate).

ALTERNATIVE DECISION CRITERIA

Strictly following the standard EMV approach, you pick the choice with the highest *average* payoff from its set of terminal events. By this standard, apply-MSW is the best choice.

A different criterion is *maximin*. Pick the course with the "best worst outcome." That is, the choice whose *worst* alternative is highest. If one choice offered a range of payoffs from $1,000 gain to $500 loss, and another a range of +$300 to +100, maximin chooses the second one. This is a defensive choice, sacrificing highest average payoff for security, like putting your money in treasury bonds versus more profitable but riskier stocks. "A bird in the hand is worth any number in the bush." In our example, the maximin choice is not to apply at all, guaranteeing a return of at least $400,000 as compared with the $370,000 of accept-drop for either MSW or PhD.

At the opposite extreme is *maximax*, which picks the choice with the highest *best*-case payoff, regardless of the odds. In our illustration, this choice is to go for the PhD. Lottery players do this in their pursuit of a multi-million-dollar payoff, even though the odds are stacked to return only about half the proceeds as winnings. On a more calculated basis, this is the choice of bold entrepreneurs. It may also be a rational approach for desperate circumstances: "Workers of the world unite! You have nothing to lose but your chains."

Many people are drawn nonrationally in a direction of maximax by wishful thinking, convinced in their hearts their odds are better than the decision tree tells them, as in Garrison Keillor's Lake Wobegon, where "all the children are above average." Hey, why play games? These are *your* estimates. If it is wishful thinking, admit it. On the other hand, if you truly think your optimism is justified, why not recalculate average EMVs based on what you really think the probabilities are? Although the PhD program accepts only 20 percent of its applicants, a mentally healthy student at the top of her class may legitimately believe she has a 90 percent probability of acceptance. (Conversely, perhaps a middling-good student should revise her estimate downward to 10 percent.) If you are ambivalently optimistic, why not chart it twice, with a "middle" and an "optimistic" estimate, and then compare them thoughtfully?

A middle course between "min" and "max" is *sensitivity analysis*. Define your minimum tolerable outcome. Within that limitation, go for the highest probable payoff. In our example, if you can live with a $370,000 outcome, you will choose the MSW application.

Marginal utility may be a key factor in sensitivity analysis. A multimillionaire can tolerate a more negative worst case than a person with limited resources. A loss which he can shrug off would wipe you out. He can therefore afford to take higher investment risks for higher payoffs, whereas "you bet your *bottom* dollar" only on something safe.

Which criterion you use and how you apply it requires judgments which may vary significantly according to circumstances. Based on marginal utility, for instance, I have a three-tier pension investment plan. The portion of my equity pension plan on which I will depend for minimum adequacy is invested in a maximin "fixed income annuity," while the remainder, which will provide amenities, is invested in an EMV-based "variable annuity." With the security of this dual plan, maximax makes sense for a supplemental IRA.

Plan B

The decision tree is a tool, not a tyrant. You are not bound to what is on the tree. After all, who put it there? You did! What's to stop you from coming up with other possibilities?

On second thought, in the case illustration, PhD rejection need not be terminal. Its chain can be extended by a new choice fork (apply for MSW or take a job). This enhances the PhD option by incorporating, at a later choice fork, the MSW alternative which had formerly been treated as mutually exclusive. Better yet, add a fourth choice-branch to your tree—"apply to both at the same time," pursuing the MSW as a consolation prize if you don't get into the PhD. This charts out better than any of the original three choices:

FOURTH SCENARIO

		P		P	JP	Net Earnings	Share
	PHD ADMIT — .2		FINISH .6 — .12			$1,150,000	$138,000
			DROP .4 — .08			$ 370,000	$ 29,600
Dual Applic Choice Branch	PHD REJECT/ MSW ADMIT — .6		FINISH .9	.54		$ 700,000	$378,000
			DROP .1	.06		$ 370,000	$ 22,200
	BOTH REJECT .2			.20		$ 400,000	$120,000
Average EMV		(1.0)		(1.00)			**$647,800**

But wait, there may be yet a fifth scenario to be found: a post-Master's PhD program which counts MSW credits toward its degree. It extends the MSW graduation chain beyond its former terminal event to a new choice fork (apply to go on for the PhD or not). About 50 percent of my MSW graduates who later apply to PhD programs are accepted, of which 80 percent graduate. Thus, they can have their cake and eat it too: the security of the MSW plus a 40 percent chance to go on to the PhD salary level if they choose. This may be the best average EMV payoff of all.

The message? Don't stop thinking just because you have done one decision-tree scenario. Maybe there is a still better scenario waiting in the wings for you to discover it.

PROS AND CONS

Stochastic decision analysis can greatly improve informed choice. It can be plugged into whatever empirical or estimated data you can muster. By breaking it down step-by-step, a complex set of uncertainties are addressed one at a time, then put together to provide an overall view. It is consistent, applying the same values, assumptions, and external realities throughout. It is capable of considering all outcomes and usually does so for each "finalist" course of action. Finally, it can stimulate creativity. Especially when the planner is not fully satisfied with any of his or her options, this strategic overview of the layout of interrelated factors may encourage the planner to come up with something better than any of the original choices, as in the case of our illustration's fourth and fifth scenarios above.

On the other side, it has the perennial GIGO risk. The soundness of the decision tree, however perfectly executed, is only as good or as bad as the accuracy of its estimates of probability and its pricing of the EMV.

Then there is the danger of becoming myopic in the course of decomposition. Theoretically you don't, because you break it down within a clear overall framework and put it back together at the end. In practice, this rather mechanistic process can reduce our holistic gestalt vision, causing us to lose the "feel of the road."

Where subjective guesstimates are used, getting consensus on them can be difficult, except in small-scale planning or where there is an accepted arbiter, such as the boss.

When is it most useful? When you know enough to make good projections on outcome values and probabilities. When you want a single overview perspective that covers both desirability (EV) and feasibility (P). This may be in most projects.

Is there a time when it may *not* be useful? Yes: an unstable environment in which you can't make reliable predictions, such as intense political conflict, an economic crisis, or arbitrary and capricious superiors. If you can't predict, you can't calculate probability.

REFERENCE

Coyle, R. (1972). *Decision analysis*. London: Nelson.

Epilogue

Planning as Social Practice

This book has identified a variety of possible ways of thinking, approaches to planning, ethical and value choices, models, general methods, and specific techniques. Nobody is truly "objective" or "detached." However, within the limits of my own slants, I have tried to present the assets and liabilities of each as fairly as I reasonably could. Now, here in this epilogue, are my personal views on planning.

TO WHAT END?

If you don't know where you are going, you probably won't get there. If you are lucky, you will get nowhere in particular. Worse, you may end up someplace you wish you weren't.

Planning is a means to an end. You can't plan without a destination. Incredibly, this aspect is given short shrift in most planning, which tends to start with specific objectives or, at most, five-year intermediate goals. A notable exception is "strategic management" which always begins with a review of the organization's *mission statement.* Unfortunately, even this tends to be incrementalist in practice, with little if any nonbounded soul searching.

I cannot stress enough the global vision and VIBES perspective as a prerequisite to good social planning. We must know where we are going **and why.**

This means having a perspective on ultimate ends. To what purpose? What is the desirable situation we are aiming toward, even if it is not fully achievable, and why is it desirable? What are our key premises and assumptions (especially values and beliefs about reality) on which it is based? Where are we coming from, both figuratively and literally? What is our vantage point–in tradition, culture, educational slants, religion, historical perspective, ideology, class, and reference groups?

It is impossible not to have these biases. The pseudo-objectivity of positivism, classical science, and the "pure" classical CRAM model is either self-deception or cynically self-serving. (It is easier to confront a conscious evil than a misguided good intentions.)

It's okay to have slants. Everybody does. Don't apologize for them. What is important is to be aware of them, modify them if appropriate, affirm them. Make sure they are "good" slants, what Gadamer (1975) calls, "true prejudices." Acknowledge them openly to yourself and, unless there are specific strategic reasons for not doing so, to others.

To the extent that our planning affects others (targets and stakeholders), it is ethically desirable to know as much as possible about their VIBES too. Strategically, it is equally important to know the VIBES of those who can affect the success of our planning (actors). Sometimes these are the same people.

From this solid base are derived all other goals, objectives, and means. Strategic goals must contribute toward the desirable situation. Objectives must explicitly achieve a piece of the goal or be a stepping-stone toward doing so, and not preclude further progress. Means must be compatible with ultimate goals and VIBES, and not subvert them.

Without this perspective, planning can go awry. A classic example was the Family Assistance Plan (FAP) of the early 1970s. Its originator, a White House aide, Daniel Moynihan, conceived it as a bold antipoverty program to assure minimum adequacy for poor children and their mothers. Faced with a diversity of state AFDC (Aid to Families with Dependent Children) programs which ranged from near the official poverty line to as little as $10 per person per month, he proposed a goal of a single universal national family assistance program with adequate living grants plus training and work experience services to help parents get off welfare. By the time it had been compromised with President Nixon and two houses of Congress, it had become a plan to save money through an efficient and thrifty national program which carried a grant level below what 70 percent of the families were already receiving. It excluded more poor families than before, and substituted "free" punitive threats for expenditures on developmental services. Its effect would have been to *increase* poverty rather than reduce it. The planner castigated his earlier allies for organizing to defeat his final plan, but they saw what he himself missed: in his eagerness to achieve a national AFDC, he had compromised away its original intent.

Similarly, academic programs, in pursuit of the laudable objective of increasing faculty "scholarly production" may set up an implementation design (e.g., salary, promotion, and tenure incentives and sanctions) which subverts its primary mission of producing the best possible professional practitioners. Or a student may pursue the desirable goal of a professional education to improve one's quality of life at a work and stress overload level which damages his or her long-term health and family life interests.

Balancing Desirability and Feasibility

There is also a flip side. The finest therapeutic or social goal does my client, agency, or community no good if nothing comes of it. In her autobiography, Agatha Christie (1977) observed,

> It is not good writing a novel of thirty thousand words–that is not a length which is easily publishable at present. If you want to write a book, study what sizes books are and write within the limits of that size. If you want to write a certain type of short story for a certain type of magazine, you have to make it the length, and it has to be the type of story, that is printed in that magazine. If you like to write for yourself, that is a different matter–you can make it any length, and write it in any way you wish; but then you will probably have to be content with the pleasure alone of having written it.

Don't become so heavenly minded that you're no earthly good. In this best of all possible worlds, we can rarely achieve an ideal goal without compromise. The larger the plan, the more people are involved as actors and stakeholders, the more compromise and accommodation will be required.

Somehow, we must find an uneasy compromise between the

desirable and the feasible. This theme appears repeatedly throughout the book in nearly every chapter. There are few clear answers. For me, and perhaps for you, it is the hardest part of planning.

DON'T BE A ONE-NOTE CHARLIE

If you want to do a poor planning job, use one way of thinking, one type of data, one model, one technique. Nearly every one of those discussed in this book has merit in its place and within its limitations. None is totally reliable by itself.

The chapter on systems models and worldviews presents a variety of them because each has its particular assets. The same is true of the section on different approaches to planning. In the first assignment of my planning course, students compare the similarities and differences between any two different planning approaches they choose and then give their personal views on either (1) how to combine the best of both into a synthesis which is better than either alone, or (2) when they would use one and when the other, depending on the particular planning purpose and circumstances. Some of their observations are included in this book. I usually find myself using different systems models, ways of thinking, general approaches, and techniques at different levels or stages within any given plan.

Particularly important is to incorporate both quantitative and qualitative, tangible and intangible, empirical and intuitional elements. I may start with "hard" data or with experience-based insight, with research findings or with hunches. Whichever I start with, I always try to check it against the other. Check your findings against your gut feelings, and your intuition against hard data.

Economic measures are extremely useful, both for the information they give you and as an aid to persuading others. But never rely totally on the economic, for "the best things is life are free." Well, maybe not free, but certainly the highest human values and satisfactions cannot be measured in dollars alone. At the same time, economics, if not an end in itself, is one of the most important means available to achieve human purposes.

By the same token, don't rely on only one kind of data. No single source is without bias, selectiveness, omissions, and distortion.

Rely on multiple sources, including a mix of empirical studies, refined theory, personal experience (yours and others'), anecdotal accounts, and journalism, as well as insightful expressions in essays, drama, fiction, and other art mediums. This does not assure you of objective Truth, but it may get you as close as you can get—hopefully close enough for you to plan and achieve something good.

PLANNING IS A TOOL, NOT AN END IN ITSELF

This book has provided a BASIC, generic planning model and a variety of techniques for elaborating and selecting goals, scheduling and managing implementation, assessing needs, defining results, putting a value on inputs and outputs, involving stakeholders, calculating unknowns, estimating risks, handling unexpected contingencies, etc.

These techniques are the distillation of many creative people based on their extensive practice experience. It is wise to know them and use them. Many of them are sophisticated, entailing advanced mathematics, social research methods, technological formulae, hardware, and software.

Not a few planning programs teach and prescribe them as essential to orthodoxy. They are right, to a significant extent. For certain specific settings and tasks, anything less is a regrettable compromise. From this book you should have a good awareness of what they are, what they do, what they are good for, what they are not good for, when to use them, and, at a beginning level, how to use them.

However, they are not idols to worship. They are tools: no more, no less. In real life, you will select your tools and, inevitably, cut corners.

There may be more than one way to skin a cat. How do I handle the fall leaves in my large yard with its many trees? Well, I can rake, mow and bag, blow, or mulch. These have different costs, involve more or less manual work, and have better or worse ecological side effects. (My neighbor used a default approach: he did nothing and called his yard a "lovely rustic setting.") For your planning yard, you may use a choice of tools, a mix of them, or, like my neighbor, choose the default alternative.

You may know better how to do something than available time, resources, and expertise permit. I also have a large driveway to shovel in winter. My neighbor had a snow blower, but I couldn't afford one, so I bought a good shovel. It took longer and was more work (which I claimed was "great exercise"), but I achieved the same end. Later, I had the money to buy one myself, but alas, they were sold out and no more would be ordered until next fall. So I continued to shovel. No sweat! (Oops, a poor metaphor; how about "no big deal!")

The message: if you can't do your planning as well as you want to, do the best job you can with the tools at hand. Maybe in the future you can afford the snow blower. Meanwhile, shoveling is better than being snowed in (I keep telling myself).

Then there is the Law of Parsimony. Do however much is sufficient for the task. Anything more than that is a waste. Don't use a steam shovel to dig a hole for your azalea bush. On the other hand, don't use a spade to dig the foundation for an office building.

There are exceptions to the Law. As we have seen with needs assessment, your planning effort may also perform secondary functions which warrant doing more than "enough." Several of my students who did much more than required on their course planning projects have parlayed them into significant career advancement. Like many of you, I often do more than necessary for my own satisfaction, learning, and self-esteem.

In 1966, I served on a DHEW task force to develop PPBS (a cost benefit analysis system) for federal human services. The real brains of the task force was a young woman name Alice Rivlin. She put together a great cost-benefit analysis system (within the limits discussed earlier in this book, of course). It was mostly wasted effort. The president who mandated it continued to make his decisions on an intuitive gut level. Congress paid little attention to it, pursuing business as usual with lobbyists, special interests, and squeaky wheels. The next president rescinded it altogether. However, for the next thirty years, the expertise and insight she gained in the process contributed to the immense respect and influence she carried as head of the Congressional Budget Office and later as Director of the United States Office of Budget and Management.

Still, for the most part, you can take all this good planning stuff and use its basic concepts and methods modestly to give you a major step forward from not planning. As I tell my students, the most important goal of the course is to develop a habit of thinking in a systematic planning way. The skills and techniques they learn are "profit."

This "planning habit," once acquired, should enhance your personal future, casework, treatment plans, agency programming, community organization, teaching, doing research projects, and every other phase of life that can benefit from thinking ahead with perspective.

THE BOTTOM LINE

When the smoke clears, the bottom line of all policy and planning, as of all social work and human service practice, is whether any real person (individual) is better off as a result of your course of action.

> He who would do good to another must do it in Minute Particulars.
> General Good is the Plea of the scoundrel, hypocrite, and flatterer;
> for Art and Science cannot exist but in minutely organized particulars.

—William Blake
"Jerusalem," *1811*

REFERENCE

Christie, A. (1977). *Agatha Christie: An autobiography.* New York: Ballentine.
Gadamer, H. (1975). *Truth and method.* 4th ed. New York: Seabury.

Bibliography

GENERAL PLANNING METHODS AND MODELS

Bassett, E. (1938). *The master plan.* New York: Russell Sage.

Bauer, R. & Gergen, K. (Eds.) (1968). *The study of policy formation.* London: Collier Macmillan.

Bennis W., Benne, K., & Chin, R. (1985). *The planning of change.* 4th ed. New York: Holt, Rinehardt & Winston.

Bennis, W. (1990). *Why leaders can't lead.* San Francisco: Jossey Bass.

Bicanic, R. (1967). *Problems of planning East and West.* Hague: Mouton.

Branch, M. (1990). *Planning: Universal process.* New York: Praeger.

Bruton, M. (Ed.) (1974). *The spirit and purpose of planning.* London: Hutchison.

Burchell, R. & Sternlieb, G. (Eds.) (1979). *Planning theory in the 1980s.* New Brunswick: Center for Urban Policy Research.

Capra, F. (1984). *The tao of physics.* 2nd ed. New York: Bantam.

Cherry, G. (1974). "The development of planning thought." In Bruton, M. (Ed.), *The spirit and purpose of planning.* London: Hutchinson.

Cowan, P. (1979). *The future of planning.* London: Heinemann.

Dluhy, M. & Chen, K. (Eds.) (1986). *Interdisciplinary planning.* New York: Center for Urban Planning.

Drucker, P. (1959). *Long range planning. Mgmt Sciences,* 4.

Dyckman, J. (1979). "Three crises in American planing." In Burchell, R. & Sternlieb, G. (Eds.), *Planning theory in the 1980s.* New Brunswick: Center for Urban Policy Research.

Faludi, A. (Ed.) (1973). *A reader in planning theory.* New York: Pergamon.

Fayol, H. (1916). *General and industrial management.* (English edition, 1949; London: Pitman.)

Gilbert, N. & Specht, H. (Eds.) (1977). *Planning for social welfare.* Englewood Cliffs, NJ: Prentice Hall.

Gleick, J. (1987). *Chaos: Making a new science.* New York: Penguin.

Howard, E. (1902). *Garden cities of tomorrow.* (Reprint, 1965; London: Faber & Faber.)

International City Management Association (1988). *The practice of local government planning.* 2nd ed., ICMA, Washington, D.C.

Kahn, A. (1969). *Theory and practice of social planning.* New York: Russell Sage.

Kohl, H. (1992). *From archetype to zeitgeist.* Boston: Little Brown.

Lindblom, C. (1968). *The policy making process.* Englewood Cliffs, NJ: Prentice Hall.

Machiavelli, N. (1537). *The prince.*

Mayer, R. (1985). *Policy and program planning: A developmental perspective.* Englewood Cliffs, NJ: Prentice-Hall.

McGuire, C. and Radnor, R. (1987). *Decision and organization.* Amsterdam: N Holland, pp. 161-176.

Rothman J. & Toler, M. (1986). "Planning theory and planning practice." In Dluhy, M. and Chen, K. (Eds.), *Interdisciplinary planning.* New York: Center for Urban Planning.

Shafritz, J. & Ott, S. (1987). *Classics of organizational theory.* 2nd ed. Chicago: Dorsey.

Simon, H. (1972). "Theories of Bounded Rationality." In McGuire, C. & Radnor, R. (Eds.), *Decision and organization.* Amsterdam: N Holland.

Smith, J. & Rade, N. (1988). "Rational and non-rational planning." *Long Range Planning,* 4.

Soule, G. (1967). *Planning USA.* New York: Viking.

Taylor, F. (1916). *Principles of scientific management.* New York: Harpert Brothers.

Troub, R. (1982). "A general theory of planning: The evolution of planning and the planning of evolution." *Journal of Economic Issues,* 6.

United Way of America (1974). *Program planning.* Alexandria, VA.

Wildavsky, A. (1973). "If planning is everything, maybe it's nothing." *Policy Sciences,* 4, pp. 127-153.

Zwicky, F. (1969). *Discovery, intervention, and research through the morphological approach.* New York: Macmillan.

APPROACHES

Alexander, E. (1992). *Approaches to planning.* Philadelphia: Gordon & Breach.

Altschuler, A. (1965). "The goals of comprehensive planning." *Journal of the American Institute of Planners,* 31.

Banfield, E. (1955). "Notes on a conceptual scheme." In Meyerson, M. & Banfield , E. (Eds.), *Politics, planning and the public interest.* New York: Free Press.

Berry, B. (1979). "Notes on an expedition to planland." In Burchell, R. & Steinlieb, G. (Eds.), *Planning theory in the 1980s.* New Brunswick: Center for Urban Policy Research.

Berry, D. (1974) "The transfer of planning theories to health planning practice." *Policy Sciences,* 5, pp. 343-361.

Davidoff, P. (1965). "Advocacy and pluralism in planning." *Journal of the American Institute of Planners,* 31, pp. 331-338.

Dror, Y. (1964). "Muddling through–'science' or inertia?" *Public Admin Rev,* 24.

Dror, Y. (1963). "The planning process: A facet design." *International Review of Administrative Sciences,* 29, pp. 46-58.

Etzioni, A.(1967). "Mixed scanning: A third approach to decision making." *Public Administration Review,* 27, pp. 385-392.

Etzioni, A. (1968). *The active society.* New York: Free Press.

Friedman, J. (1979). "Theory of meta-planning: Innovation, flexible response and social learning." In Burchell, R. & Sternlieb, G. (Eds.), *Planning theory in the 1980s.* New Brunswick: Center for Urban Policy Research.

Hudson, B. (1979). "Comparisons of current planning theories." *Journal of the American Institute of Planners,* 45, pp. 387-398.

Lindblom, C. (1959). "The science of muddling through." *Public Admin Review,* 19, pp. 79-88.

Lindblom, C. (1979). "Still muddling, not yet through." *Public Admin Review,* 39, pp. 517-526.

McConkey, D. (1974). *Management by results.* New York: ANACOM.

Meyerson, M. & Banfield, E. (1955). *Politics, planning and the public interest.* New York: Free Press.

Meyerson, M. (1956). "Building the middle-range bridge for comprehensive planning." *Journal American Institute of Planners*, 22.

O'Conner, R. (1978). *Planning under uncertainty: Multiple scenarios and contingency planning.* New York: Conference Board.

Odiorne, G. (1965). *Management by objectives.* New York: Pitman.

Rein, M. (1969). "Social planning: The search for legitimacy." *Journal of the American Institute of Planners*, 35, pp. 233-244.

Rittell, H. & Webber, M. (1973). "Dilemmas of a general theory of planning." *Policy Sciences*, 4, pp. 133-145.

Sillince, J. (1986). *A theory of planning.* Brookfield, VT: Gower.

Simon, H. (1957). *Administrative behavior.* New York: Macmillan.

Simon, H. (1957). *Models of man.* New York: Wiley.

Wilson, D. (1980). *The national planning idea in US public policy: 5 alternative approaches.* Boulder: Westview.

DECISION ANALYSIS

Arrow, J. (1977). "Alternative approaches to to the theory of choice in risk-taking situations." *Econometrics*, 19, pp. 607-622.

Bower, J. (1968). "Descriptive decision theory from the administrative viewpoint." In Bauer, R. & Gergen, K. (Eds.), *The study of policy formation.* London: Collier Macmillan.

Coyle, R. (1972). *Decision analysis.* London: Nelson.

Hooker, C. et al. (Eds.) (1978). *Foundations and applications of decision theory.* 2 vols. Boston: D. Reidel.

Horn, R. & Cheaves, A. (Eds.) (1980). *The guide to simulation games.* 4th ed. Beverly Hills: Sage.

Howard, R. (1980). "An assessment of decision analysis." *Operations Research*, 28.

Keeney, R. & Raiffa, H. (1976). *Decisions with multiple objectives, preferences, and values.* New York: Wiley.

March, J. (1982). "Theories of choice and making decisions." *Transaction-Society*, 20, pp. 29-39.

Merkhofer, M. (1987). *Decision science and social risk management.* Boston: D. Reidel.

Nutt, P. (1981). "Some guides for the selection of a decision- making strategy." *Technological Forecasting and Social Change*, 19.

Pitz, G. & McKillip, J. (1984). *Decision analysis for program evaluators.* Beverly Hills: Sage.

Pratt, J., Raiffa, H., & Schlaifer, R. (1964) "The foundations of decision under uncertainty." *Journal of American Statistical Association*, 59, pp. 353-375.

Radford, K. (1977). *Complex decision problems: An integrated strategy for their resolution.* Reston: Reston Publishing Co.

Raiffa, H. & Schlaifer R. (1961). *Applied statistical decision theory.* Cambridge: Harvard.

Rycus, M. (1982). *Decision analysis.* Stroudsburg: Hutchison Ross.

Tropman, J. (1981). "Value conflicts and decision making: Analysis and resolution." *Community Development Journal*, 16.

Von Neumann, J. & Morgenstern, O. (1947). *Theories of games and economic behavior.* Princeton: Princeton Univ.

Watson, S. (1979). *Decision analysis as a replacement for cost benefit analysis.* Cambridge [UK]: CUED, F-CAMS, TR197.

Zagare, F. (1984). *Game theory: Concepts and applications.* Beverly Hills: Sage.

Zeleny, M. (19822). *Multiple criteria decision making.* New York: McGraw-Hill.

ECONOMICS AND OTHER QUANTIFICATION METHODS

Anderson, L. & Settle, R. (1977). *Benefit-cost analysis: A practice guide.* Lexington, MA: Lexington.

Augustinovics, M. (1975). *Integration of mathematics and traditional methods of planning.* In Bornstein, M. (Ed.), *Economic planning: East and West.* Cambridge, MA: Ballinger.

Beauregard, R. (1979). *Planning in an advanced capitalist state.* In Burchell, R. & Sternlieb, G. (Eds.), *Planning theory in the 1980s.* New Brunswick: Center for Urban Policy Research.

Bentham, J. (1823/1948). *An introduction to the principles of morals and legislation.* New York: Hafner.

Bornstein, M. (Ed.) (1975) *Economic planning: East and West.* Cambridge, MA: Ballinger.

deGraaf, J. (1957). *Theoretical welfare economics.* Cambridge: Cambridge University.

Frantz, R. (1988). *X-efficiency: Theory, evidence and applications.* Boston: Kluwer.

Hapgood, F. (1979). "Risk-benefit analysis: Putting a price on life." *Atlantic*, Vol. 243, No. 1, pp. 33-38.

Haverman, R. & Margolis, J. (Eds.) (1970). *Public expenditures and policy analysis.* Chicago: Marckham.

Hicks, J. (1943). "The four consumer surpluses." *Review of Economic Studies,* Vol. II, No.1, pp. 31-41.

Kaldor, N. (1939). "Welfare propositions in economics." *Economic Journal.* Vol. 49, pp. 549-552.

Kume, H. (1985). *Statistical methods for quality improvement.* Tokyo: 3A Corp.

Levin, H. (1983). *Cost effectiveness, a primer.* Beverly Hills: Sage.

Liebenstein, H. (1989). *Essays [on X-efficiency].* New York: New York Univ.

Little, I. (1957). *A critique of welfare economics.* Oxford: Oxford Press.

Lowi, T. (1970). "Decision making versus policy making: toward an antidote for technocracy." *Public Administration Review,* 30, pp. 314-325.

Mills, H.(1959). *Mathematics and the managerial imagination.* Princeton: Mathematica.

Mishan, E. (1976). *Cost-benefit analysis.* 2nd ed. New York: Praeger.

Pareto, V. (1909). *Manuel d'economique politique.* Paris: M. Girard.

Peacock, A. (1973). *Cost benefit analysis and the control of public expenditure.* In Wolfe, J. (Ed.), *Cost benefit and cost effectiveness.* London: Allen & Unwind.

Pearce, D. (1983). *Cost benefit analysis.* London: Macmillan.

Pigou, A. (1932). *The economics of welfare.* London: MacMillan.

Rivlin, A. (1970). *The program planning and budgeting system in DHEW: Some lessons from experience.* In Haverman, R. & Margolis, J. (Eds.), *Public expenditures and policy analysis.* Chicago: Markham.

Rivlin, A. (1971). *Systematic thinking for social action.* Washington: Brookings.

Sassene, P. (1978). *Cost benefit analysis: A handbook.* New York: Academic Press.

Self, P. (1975). *Econocrats and the policy process*. London: Macmillan.

Slaybaugh, C. (1966). "Pareto's law and modern management." *Waterhouse Review*, Winter, 1966.

Wildavsky, A. (1975). *Budgeting: A comparative theory of budgetary processes*. Boston: Little Brown.

Wolfe, J. (Ed.) (1973). *Cost benefit and cost effectiveness*. London: Allen & Unwind.

Zeckhauser, R. et al., (Eds.) (1974). *Benefit-cost and policy analysis*. Chicago: Aldine.

NEEDS ASSESSMENT

Burch, G. (1981). *Assessment of primary health care needs of north and south Omaha*. Omaha: Univ of Nebraska.

Johnson, D. (1987). *Needs assessment: Theory and methods*. Ames: Iowa State.

Lauffer, A. (1982). *Assessment tools*. Beverly Hills: Sage.

League of California Cities (1975). *Assessing human needs*. Sacramento.

McKillip, J. (1987). *Need analysis*. Newbury Park: Sage.

Neuber, K. (1980). *Needs Assessment*. Beverly Hills: Sage.

Siemiatycki, J. (1979). "A comparison of mail, telephone, and home interview strategies for household health surveys." *American Journal of Public Health*, 69.

United Way of America. (1982). *Needs Assessment*. Alexandria, VA.

Warheit G., Bell, R., & Schwab, J. (1977). *Needs assessment approaches: Concepts and methods*. U.S. Govt, DHEW, Publication #(ADM)77-472.

PARTICIPATION

Alinsky, S. (1972). *Rules for radicals*. New York: Vintage.

Arnstein, S. (1969). "A ladder of citizen participation." *Journal of the American Institute of Planners*, 35, pp. 216-224.

Boone, R. (1972). "Reflections on citizen participation and the Economic Opportunity Act." *Public Administration Review*, 32, pp. 444-456.

Cloward, R. & Ohlin, L. (1960). *Delinqency and opportunity.* New York: Free Press.

Dalky, N. (1967). *Delphi.* Santa Monica: Rand.

Davidoff, P. (1979). *The redistribution function in planning: Creating greater eqality among citizens of communities.* In Burchell R. & Steinlieb, G. (Eds.), *Planning theory in the 1980s.* New Brunswick: Center for Urban Policy Research.

Delbecq, A. & Van de Ven, A. (1971). "A group process model for problem identification." *Journal of Applied Behavioral Science,* 7, pp. 466-492.

Delbecq, A. et al. (1975). *Group techniques for program planning: A guide to nominal group and delphi processes.* Glenview: Scott Foresman.

Fisher, R. & Ury, W. (1981). *Getting to YES.* New York: Penguin.

Friedman, J. (1973). *Retracking America: A theory of transactive planning.* New York: Doubleday.

Industrial Areas Foundation (1990). *IAF 50 years: Organizing for change.* New York: Franklin Square.

Kahn, S. (1991). *Organizing.* Silver Spring, MD: NASW/1991.

Kasperson, R. & Breitbart, M. (1974). *Participation, decentralization, and advocacy planning,* Washington: Association of American Geographers.

Lauffer, A. (1978). *Social planning at the community level.* Englewood cliffs: Prentice Hall.

Peattie, L. (1968). Reflections on advocacy planning. *Journal of the American Institute of Planners,* 34, pp. 80-88.

Rubin, L. (1967). "Maximum feasible participation: The origins, implications, and present status." *Poverty & Human Resources Abstracts,* 2.

Selznick, P. (1949). *TVA and the grass roots: Democracy on the march.* Berkeley: U. of California.

PROJECT MANAGEMENT/PERT

Archibald, R. (1987). "The history of modern project management: Key milestones in early PERT/CPM/PDM days." *Project Management Journal,* 18, pp. 9-31.

Canada, Government: Regional and Economic Expansion (1982). *Project management handbook*. Ottawa.

Fondahl, J. (1987). "The history of modern project management." *Project Management Journal,* 18, pp. 33-36.

Jackman, H. (1990). "State of the art project management methods: a survey." *Optimum*, 20, pp. 24-47.

Johnson, G (1987). "Expediting projects in PERT with stochastic time estimates." *Project Management Journal*, 21, pp. 29-34.

Mulvaney, J. (1975). *Analysis bar charting*. Washington, DC: Management Planning and Control Systems.

Shelmerdine, E. (1989). "Planning for project management." *Journal of Systems Management*, 40, pp. 16-20.

STRATEGIC PLANNING APPROACHES

Barra, R. (1989). *Putting quality circles to work*. New York: McGraw Hill.

Bryson, J. (1988). *Strategic planning for public and nonprofit organizations*. San Francisco: Jossey Bass.

Crosby, P. (1985). *Quality without tears*. New York: Plume.

Deming, W. E. (1986). *Out of crisis*. Cambridge, MA: MIT.

Hart, S. (1986). "Planning as a strategic social process." In Dluhy M. & Chen, K. (Eds.), *Interdisciplinary planning*. New York: Center for Urban Planning.

Imai, M. (1986). *Kaizen*. New York: Random House.

Koontz, H. (1972). *Principles of management: an analysis of managerial functions*. 5th ed. New York: McGraw Hill.

Koteen, J. (1989). *Strategic management in public and nonprofit organizations*. New York: Praeger.

Mason, R. & Mitroff, D. (1981). *Challenging stragegic planning assumptions*. New York: Wiley.

Senge, P (1990). *The 5th discipline*. New York: Doubleday.

Steiner, G. (1979). *Strategic planning*. New York: Free Press.

Taylor, B. (1984). "Strategic planning: Which style do you need?" *Long Range Planning*, 4.

Tenner, A. & DeToro, I. (1992). *Total quality management*. Reading, MA: Addison-Wesley.

Thompson, A. & Strickland, A. (1989) *Strategic formulation and implementation.* 4th ed. Homewood, IL: Irwin.

Walter, S. & Choate, P. (1984). *Thinking and acting strategically.* Washington: Council of State Planning Agencies.

Walton, M. (1986). *The Deming management method.* New York: Dodd Mead.

SYSTEMS AND PLANNING

Ackoff, R. (Ed.) (1974). *Systems and management annual.* New York: Petrocelli.

Bailey, J. (1975). *Social theory for planning.* London: Routledge & Kegan Paul.

Baker (1973). *Organizatinal Systems.* Homewood, IL: R.D. Irwin.

Bertalanffy L. von. (1974). "The history and status of general systems theory." In Ackoff, R. (Ed.), *Systems and management annual.* New York: Petrocelli.

Bertalanffy, L. von. (1975). *Perspectives on general systems theory.* New York: George Braziller.

Boulding, K. (1956). "General systems theory." *Management Science Journal,* 2, pp. 244-250.

Churchman, C. W. (1979). *The systems approach and its enemies.* New York: Basic Books.

Hughes, J. & Mann L. (1969). "Systems and planning theory." *Journal of American Institute of Planners,* 35, pp. 330-33

Parsons, T. (1950). *The social system.* Glencoe, IL: Free Press.

Rapoport, A. (1968). *General systems theory.* In Silk, D. (Ed.), *International encyclopedia of the social sciences.* Vol. 15. New York: Macmillan.

Roges, C. (1989). In H. Kirschbaum and V. Henderson (Eds.), *The Carl Rogers Reader.* Boston: Houghton Mifflin.

Silk, D. (Ed.) (1968). *International encyclopedia of the social sciences.* Vol. 15. New York: Macmillan.

VALUES AND ETHICS

Boulding, K. (1966). "The ethics of rational decision." *Management Science Journal,* 12, p.161.

Burch, H. (1991). *The whys of policy.* New York: Praeger.

Davidoff, P & Reiner, T. (1962). "A choice theory of planning." *Journal of the American Institute of Planners*, 28, pp. 103-15.

Dunn, W. (Ed.) (1983). *Values, ethics and the practice of policy analysis.* Lexington, MA: DC Heath.

Gadamer, H. (1975). *Truth & method.* 4th ed. New York: Seabury.

Habermas, J. (1987). *The philosophical discourse on modernity.* Cambridge, MA: MIT Press.

Mannheim, K. (1949). *Ideology and utopia.* New York: Harcourt & Brace.

Meehan, E. (1990). *Ethics for policy making: A methodological analysis.* New York: Greenwood.

Miller, S. & Riesman, F. (1968). *Social change and social planning.* New York: Basic Books.

National Conference of Catholic Bishops (1986). *Economic justice for all.* Washington.

Niebuhr, R. (1968). *Faith and politics.* New York: G. Braziller

Rawls, J. (1971). *A theory of justice.* Cambridge: Harvard.

Rein, M. (1976). *Social sciences and public policy.* New York: Penguin.

Schumacher, E. (1973). *Small is beautiful.* London: Blond.

Singer, P. (1979). *Practical ethics.* Cambridge: Cambridge Univ.

Vickers, G. (1970). *Value systems and social progress.* Baltimore: Penguin.

Warren, R. (1977). *Social change and human purpose.* Chicago: Rand McNally.

Index

OTHER TITLES AVAILABLE FROM
HAWORTH SOCIAL WORK PRACTICE

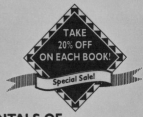

TAKE
20% OFF
ON EACH BOOK!

Special Sale!

ENVIRONMENTAL PRACTICE IN THE HUMAN SERVICES
Integration of Micro and Macro Roles, Skills, and Contexts
Bernard Neugeboren, PhD
Points to the need for the human services to return to their historic mission of environmental change.
$49.95 hard. ISBN: 1-56024-944-7. (Outside US/Canada: $60.00)
$22.95 soft. ISBN: 0-7890-6025-6. (Outside US/Canada: $28.00)
Available Spring 1996. 322 pp. plus Index.

BASIC SOCIAL POLICY AND PLANNING
Strategies and Practice Methods
Hobart A. Burch, PhD
A comprehensive introduction to policy and planning approaches, methods, models, ways of thinking, and techniques.
$39.95 hard. ISBN: 0-7890-6026-4. (Outside US/Canada/Mexico: $48.00)
Text price (5+ copies): $19.95. (Outside US/Canada/Mexico: $24.00)
Available Spring 1996. Approx. 341 pp. with Index.

SOCIAL WORK INTERVENTION IN AN ECONOMIC CRISIS
The River Communities Project
Martha Baum, PhD, and Pamela Twiss, PhD
A carefully documented study of a true experience of an area-wide economic disaster.
$29.95 hard. ISBN: 0-7890-6036-1. (Outside US/Canada/Mexico: $36.00)
Text price (5+ copies): $19.95. (Outside US/Canada/Mexico: $24.00)
Available Summer 1996. Approx. 175 pp. plus Index.

THE RELATIONAL SYSTEMS MODEL FOR FAMILY THERAPY
Living in the Four Realities
Donald R. Bardill, PhD, MSW
Provides a particular worldview for the conduct of family therapy.
$34.95 hard. ISBN: 0-7890-0074-1. (Outside US/Canada: $42.00)
Text price (5+ copies): $24.95. (Outside US/Canada: $30.00)
Available Summer 1996. Approx. 286 pp. with Index.

FEMINIST THEORIES AND SOCIAL WORK
Approaches and Applications
Christine Flynn Saulnier, PhD
Counteracts the notion of feminist theory as a single theory with multiple contradictions.
$29.95 hard. ISBN: 1-56024-945-5. (Outside US/Canada/Mexico: $37.00)
Text price (5+ copies): $19.95. (Outside US/Canada/Mexico: $24.00)
Available Summer 1996. Approx. 242 pp. with Index.

FUNDAMENTALS OF COGNITIVE-BEHAVIOR THERAPY
From Both Sides of the Desk
Bill Borcherdt
Provides a storehouse of practical, hands-on tactics that encourages problem solving.
$34.95 hard. ISBN: 0-7890-6030-2. (Outside US/Canada/Mexico:$42.00)
Text price (5+ copies): $17.95. (Outside US/Canada/Mexico: $22.00)
Available Spring 1996. Approx. 185 pp. with Index.

THE BLACK ELDERLY
Satisfaction and Quality of Later Life
Marguerite Coke, DSW and James A. Twaite, PhD, EdD
Presents the results of an empirical study of factors that influence the well-being of older black Americans.
$29.95 hard. ISBN: 1-56024-914-5. (Outside US/Canada/Mexico:$36.00)
Text price (5+ copies): $14.95. (Outside US/Canada/Mexico: $18.00)
1995. 126 pp. with Index.

THE CROSS-CULTURAL PRACTICE OF CLINICAL CASE MANAGEMENT IN MENTAL HEALTH
Edited by Peter Manoleas, MSW
Discover a culturally competent model of clinical case management for mental health practitioners.
$29.95 hard. ISBN: 1-56024-874-2. (Outside US/Canada/Mexico:$36.00)
Text price (5+ copies): $19.95. (Outside US/Canada/Mexico: $24.00)
1995. 232 pp.

FAMILY BEYOND FAMILY
The Surrogate Parent in Schools and Other Community Agencies
Sanford Weinstein, EdD, MSW
A guide for educators and others in human services seeking to bring order and meaning to chaotic lives.
$49.95 hard. ISBN: 1-56024-442-9. (Outside US/Canada: $60.00)
Text price (5+ copies): $19.95. (Outside US/Canada/Mexico: $24.00)
1995. 233 pp. with Index.

PEOPLE WITH HIV AND THOSE WHO HELP THEM
Challenges, Integration, Intervention
R. Dennis Shelby, PhD
This new guidebook uses the reported experiences of HIV-positive men to chart the course of living with HIV.
$39.95 hard. ISBN: 1-56024-922-6. (Outside US/Canada/Mexico: $48.00)
$14.95 soft. ISBN: 1-56023-865-8. (Outside US/Canada/Mexico: $18.00)
1995. 245 pp. with Index.

Faculty: Textbooks are available for classroom adoption consideration on a 60–day examination basis. You will receive an invoice payable within 60 along with the book. **If you decide to adopt the book, your invoice will be cancelled.** Please write to us on your institutional letterhead, indicating the textbook you would like to examine as well as the following information: course title, current text, enrollment, and decision date. *(See order form on reverse side)*

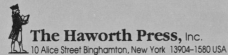

The Haworth Press, Inc.
10 Alice Street Binghamton, New York 13904–1580 USA

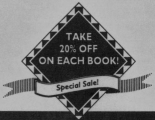